A Layman's Handbook on the Study of Natural Alternatives For a Healthy Life.

By
Dr. Randall Aiken N.D.

Seniram Publishing
Glenside, Pennsylvania 19038

Library of Congress Control Number 2012934044
ISBN #978-0-922564-04-0
Printed in the USA

Randall Aiken
3003 Mt. Carmel Ave.
Glenside, Pennsylvania 19038

Table of Contents

Preface

This book is a guide for all those who hold some curiosity about the ancient art of natural healing. However, the premise of the book does not purport to imply that mainstream medicine should be shunned, nor does it suggest that mainstream medicine does not work; rather, it is based on the findings of Doctor Samuel Hahneman, who is known as the founder of Homeopathic medicine, which he pioneered during his lifetime.

With rare exceptions, most people strive to become and remain healthy during their lifetimes. Nevertheless, for some, the goal is achieved, the greater majority of people are unable to do so. A healthy lifestyle is paramount to achieving excellent health; however, no one is invulnerable to sickness and yet, for those who are able to recognize the signs of illness in advance, there are steps that can be taken to forestall or lessen the effects of a disease before it strikes.

This book will provide a panorama of precautionary measures, each by means of a natural, non-pharmaceutical remedy. In addition, the book also outlines safe measures to be taken to combat an illness after it strikes. However, the actions are not to be considered as being prescribed; rather, they are remedies that have been prescribed by others. Each individual's body is different and the doses of the various herbs vary according to the individual. Nonetheless, examples will be clear and unambiguous as provided by professionals in the field.

It is not an obscure fact that healthcare costs in the United States has skyrocketed and there is no indication that the situation will be improving, which is why it is beneficial for everyone to compare alternatives for staying well and for the same reason to search for a natural cure; rather than depend only on pharmaceuticals that are composed of many chemicals and unnatural ingredients.

Undoubtedly, people are living longer lives as the life

expectancy continues to climb. Consumption of pharmaceuticals has escalated alarmingly, leaving some devastating side effects in its wake.

Some say that "there is not a drug that cannot be replaced with something natural." Others say that natural herbal cures are based on legends and mythology. My thoughts on the subject, concurrent with many years of studying the subject of sickness and cure, healthy and unhealthy, as well as prevention, prompted me to publish this work to provide the reader with comparisons, which will enable the reader to come to an informed decision whether to choose either a natural remedy or a pill.

The book also provides signs of various hovering illnesses and it details steps on how to read your body signals that are warnings and how to combat the threat with preemptive measures. The path to a healthy life is not difficult to travel, once you are equipped with the proper information. Many of the obstacles that block a healthy lifestyle become surmountable once you learn how to deal with them. This book will surely provide you with the proper information to place you on the fast-track to a healthy life if you conclude that you accept the challenge.

CHAPTER ONE

THE FIRST STEP
To Regain a Healthy Body

It is imperative to realize that no one can achieve a healthy body unless they receive the proper nutrients. Yet, if a body does receive the proper nutrients, but is unable to properly use the substances necessary for growth and life itself, excellent health will remain a goal that cannot be achieved. Nutrients to the body would be similar as water to a sponge. The body, like a sponge, must constantly absorb and with the body, it must absorb nutrients. Nevertheless, the process is neither complicated, nor difficult; rather, it is quite easy.

The first step requires only that you consume the proper foods, known as a balanced diet. Eating the proper food greatly supports the body's processing plant, your digestive system, which needs to be chemically balanced to properly perform its function. Chemical balance is required and must be addressed to ensure that nutrient assimilation will be 100 percent effective.

The balance is between acid and alkalinity in the blood stream, saliva and urine. It is important that the body absorbs good nutrients, which then arm the body with the ability to produce an unfriendly environment for bacteria and viruses. Ingram. E. (A reflexologist), author of *Stories Feet Can Tell.* St. Petersburg: Ingram Publishing. 2007).

For the body to effectively combat enemies, it must be alkaline, which is the way, the body was initially designed. However, the introduction of processed foods, fast-foods, carbonated soda, candy and other items has caused many people to lack proper nutrition, which in turn causes the body to be transformed from alkaline to acidic. Nonetheless, it is not only these types of food that can cause problems.

Another dangerous contributor to the cause of sickness is stress, which can alone transform an otherwise healthy body to one which becomes captive as it is transformed into acidic without any assistance from an unhealthy diet. More importantly, once stress begins to dominate the body and turn it into acidic, it becomes extremely difficult to restore the body to alkaline.

The great escalation of all types of diseases that have reached historic levels can be traced to the introduction of the previously mentioned foods. Once a person's body changes from alkaline to acidic, its defenses become vulnerable, which simultaneously causes the body to become a safe haven for bacteria, viruses and other diseases. Meanwhile, a person's body that remains alkaline through proper nutrition, retains its effective immune system, which is able to naturally combat disease. Nevertheless, it is important to remember that some organs, including the heart, pancreas, colon, kidneys and lymph glands, require more of an alkaline environment than others. Once a person has acquired a healthy body, the immune system works tirelessly to maintain good health, while often also contributing to forestalling pernicious diseases including cancer.

The balance between acid and alkalinity can easily be compared by checking your blood PH (homeostasis process). It sounds complicated; however, the process, as explained below, is simple and can be done in the privacy of your own home. Soon after, you will have an accurate measurement of your PH, which in turn will help you make the decision whether or not to begin your quest to aspire to acquire a healthy lifestyle. Once you become determined to adapt to a healthy lifestyle, you automatically begin to forestall sickness, which is not as some believe, a natural occurrence.

The method for measuring blood PH (amount of oxygen in the blood):

You will need Litmus PH test paper, which can be obtained at any health food store or you can visit to an online supplier; such as Edmunds Scientific (http://scientificsonline.com). The test papers are inexpensive and they have a very long shelf life of about two years. The test paper comes with a color chart (Green, Light Blue, Red, Blue and Dark Blue). Once the test paper is tested with either saliva or urine, you can determine your PH within about fifteen seconds, according to the color change.

The scale of the test ranges from 0-to-14, with acids ranging between 0-to-6 and alkaline from 8-to-14. When you have an alkaline measure, it indicates that your immune system is prepared to fight disease, however, in the event your acid measure is dominant, it becomes a signal that your body is lacking the proper nutrients and has become a lucrative target for disease. If you receive the warnings, do not procrastinate. Take immediate action to get yourself out of harm's way by beginning to eat properly. In conjunction, the color on the test paper will correspond to the numbered color chart, which easily identifies your count. The reading of 7.4 for saliva is considered good. Also, for urine, a good reading is 6.6.

Damage inflicted upon the body by excess acidity is not unsettled science; rather, it is a confirmed fact. In contrast, it is also widely known that the PH factor is part of the ongoing strategy to fight against and defeat diseases, including cancer. Sang Whang, the author of the book, *Reversing Aging,* expresses his thoughts on PH in the struggle against disease stated: "If your blood is to acidic, toxins will not be released from your cells into the blood. So your cells can't be detoxified. This toxic build-in cells results in acidic, poorly oxygenated cells...Degenerative diseases are the result of acid waste build-up within us." The body compensates for the acidic blood by taking minerals like calcium, magnesium, potassium and sodium from the bones and other organs to keep the body alkaline.

The dangers, caused by an over-acidic body, are sometimes identifiable early. They are poor digestion in the small intestines and the failure to properly process (metabolize) food. Poor digestion eventually leads to chronic fatigue; however, less noticeable signals include a hormonal imbalance, which can occur with both men and women when hormones (chemicals that distribute signals to the body's cells) become erratic and interfere with the body's normal activity.

The imbalance can disrupt everyday life and aggressively prevent even a good night's sleep. The imbalance can also effect a person's appetite, blood pressure, cell repair, and even growth, along with fertility and reproduction. Hormones also manage metabolism and even pain, which further underscores the necessity of eliminating an acidic body. Hormones, naturally produced throughout the body, essentially possess the ability to maintain constant communication with the body's organs and with themselves to ensure a proper balance.

Other consequences of an acidic body are more or less invisible to the naked eye, but equally pernicious. They include insufficient enzyme production, which is connected to poor digestion and it too contributes to fatigue and hormone imbalance. Yet another consequence is the lack of calcium, which causes a person's bones to decrease in density, which can cause serious problems in the event of a fall. As bone density diminishes, the solidity of a bone greatly decreases, making the bone fragile and susceptible to a fracture or break.

Other contributors to poor health due to an acidic body include an increase in insulin levels that causes a person to gain weight. However, the later attempt to lose the unwanted weight becomes a Herculean task. Neither the heart nor the muscles escape the wrath of an acidic body. Both are susceptible to damage due to insufficient amounts of electrolytes, another item that is necessary for communication between cells.

Electrolytes, including calcium, chlorine, magnesium, phosphate, potassium and sodium, are power packed minerals that literally possess an electric charge. Your body receives these minerals, which communicate with cells, from food and drink that a person consumes. These electrolytes, when unimpeded by an acidic body, contributes to a person's blood chemistry and deals primarily with the actions of a person's muscles and the heart. Electrolytes, found in the blood, urine and body fluids, contribute to maintaining proper blood chemistry. Nevertheless, when they reach dangerous low levels, serious complications can develop. Consequently, it is worthwhile to focus on attaining a healthy lifestyle to lesson the possibility of illness by initiating a steady and irrevokable balanced diet.

Assuming you are prepared to supply your body with proper nutrition to sustain alkalinity through proper dieting, other steps become necessary, because even with a strict healthy diet, your body still requires sixteen vitamins, 74 minerals and twenty-two amino acids that it must have to function properly.

These multi-vitamins and minerals are also available at health stores and online. (Chapter Three). Although the body requires proper nutrition, even those who maintain a constant balanced diet, proper levels of nutrition are not always available in food. The United States government, in an effort to inform the public of the necessity of supplementing their diets, acknowledged the importance of multi-vitamins during 1934 in a statement in the Congressional Record. It became necessary for the government to alert the public and urge that people supplement their diets with multivitamins because it had become known that over-farming the lands had greatly depleted the soil of many minerals.

Farmers now use fertilizer on the soil to grow plants with nitrogen, phosphorous and potassium. An example of a deficiency would be spinach and the myth, that by eating spinach, your body will consume all the iron it requires. Similarly, the trend continues with most foods, which is why supplemental vitamins are vital to assist in the task of maintaining a healthy body. Also, the lack of sufficient minerals in the soil is a contributing factor in the alarming number of sick people in the United States. The numbers continue to spiral upward, which coincides with the ever-rising costs of health care.

There is no cure-all that will totally eliminate illnesses; however, it is known and recommended strongly by experts in the field of medicine and health care that the paramount combination to fight sickness, both physical and mental, is first and foremost, a balanced diet. Followed with equal importance, a system of exercising, compatible with an individual's age and supplemental multi-vitamins to bolster the body's nutrients and minerals.

With regard to supplemental vitamins, the government of the United States publishes a list, known as RDAs (Recommended Daily Allowance), which provides the bare minimum of vitamins (and minerals) that the body requires on a daily basis to help prevent deficiencies and disease. See Chapter Three which provides information on vitamins and minerals that are available.

Supplements become an additional major factor in the quest to reach excellent health and it is recommended that to obtain the full complement of minerals that are not contained in multi-vitamins, you should acquire them in liquid form. A sample list of minerals is included on page 19. It is important to realize that minerals are best absorbed by the body when they are taken in liquid form.

Not surprisingly, supplementing your body's minerals and vitamins is not a complete answer. It is my opinion, based on research, that synthetically derived supplements are not totally absorbed by the body. The body is able to differentiate between natural vitamins and minerals from those that are synthetic. Consequently, an effort should always be made to acquire and consume genuine vitamins and minerals, as mentioned earlier, through diet, despite the fact that they often are elusive. Nonetheless, it is useful to buy organic foods when they are available. There are farms throughout the nation that harvest only organic foods, which are distributed to retail establishments and sold locally.

Some foods should be totally avoided. They include: white flour; white sugar, white rice, white refined salt and processed foods, all of which are detrimental to the body's armor. In contrast, a proper diet that is especially nutritious should include leafy green vegetables, fruits, grains, lean protein meats, legumes and a variety of nuts, along with substantial amounts of water.

Eating the proper foods provides great dividends. The body, through a balanced diet, receives the nutrients that power its energy and its biochemical synthesis that controls the growth of cells and tissue. In conjunction, with regard to the consumption of water as part of a balanced diet, it is recommended that a person should drink tap water; rather than bottled water. The benefits from tap water usually surpass bottled water (depending upon the water company's source of obtaining its water), primarily because it contains minerals that some bottled water does not contain.

Also, plastic bottles containing the water should be used only once and never reused due to the possibility of algae formation in the bottles. If you are a person who reuses the bottles and begin to feel tired all the time, you may have algae in your blood stream. If you find yourself with the symptom of acute tiredness, discontinue drinking water in a used bottle to allow your body to clear itself of algae.

Water is a major component of the body's cells and it is also a large part of the total weight of a body. However, many people do not consume sufficient water. Water also plays an important part in the body's ability to function properly. When the proper amount of water is contained in the body, it can reduce the level of pain from arthritis, or arthritis-like pain due to joint dehydration. The water can also prevent chapped lips, end constipation and even improve the quality of skin by helping to rid the cells of toxins.

Amazingly, the word diet, when combined with balanced, takes on a whole new responsibility and becomes the advocate or defender of a healthy body. A properly balanced diet becomes capable of surpassing medicine and it can singlehandedly rebuild the body's tissue, which medicine is incapable of accomplishing. Most importantly, disease can only be halted at the tissue level of the body. A balanced diet also permits the body to alter the course of damaged tissue to provide "wellness by increasing the efficiency and energy level of underactive glands and all internal organs, including skin, arteries, nerves and joints. (Foods That Heal Doctor, Page 12, Bernard Jensen. Avery New York, N.Y. 1988.)."

CHAPTER TWO

Detoxification

The United States, referred to as "Western Society" by many, has become a nation composed of innumerable sick people and in most cases the cause can be attributed to a poor diet and the consumption of a wide variety of food that are in great contrast to foods that provide a balanced or proper diet. The foods that contribute to an unhealthy diet include: fast foods; fried foods; processed foods; over-cooked foods and foods, particularly fruits and vegetables that are sprayed with pesticides. The consumption of improper foods causes your body to absorb unnatural substances, such as nitrates used as preservatives, antibiotics used for the health of an animal, hormones, pesticides, msg and other unknown substances (chemicals) which are approved by the FDA. These substances enter the blood stream as toxic material that causes harm to your body. The ingestion of the improper foods also prevents your body from receiving the proper nourishment that is required to maintain good health.

The human body was originally designed to consume food, while it was raw (before cooking) to ensure that all of the necessary vitamins, minerals, amino acids, enzymes and fiber were consumed. Nevertheless, in today's world, it is commonplace for food to lack fiber. Our food is usually over-processed and over-cooked, both of which essentially destroy the enzymes and nutrients. Some foods are permeated with msg, nitrates, salt, sugar and other harmful substances that are detrimental to the biological necessities of the human body, making it imperative that those foreign substances be eliminated.

In addition to the toxins in the food chain, the body is also compelled to defend against other toxins, some from the environment, such as pollution in the air, chemicals and toxic metals, along with drugs and medicines, all of which contain toxins that weaken the body's immune system to endanger your health by hindering the body's ability to fight disease.

The body's primary line of defense against toxic substances disease is three-fold, the liver, the skin and the lymph system. Nonetheless, each of the main defenders is capable only of extricating a limited amount of toxins. Consequently, once the toxins begin to overwhelm the defense system and the body becomes overloaded, the toxins pour into the bloodstream. From there, the toxins begin to rapidly search out tissue, which is located in the skin, muscles, fat and organs. Once the toxins locate the target, they initiate their pernicious task of destruction. It has been said that "the root of all disease is the "toxins in the body."

Signs of Toxification (Toxic Accumulation)--Allergies; Anxiety; Appendicitis; Arthritis; Back Aches; Bad Breath; Body Aches; Body pains; Bad Circulation; Constipation; Coughs; Depression; Dizziness; Fatigue; Fever; Frequent colds; Headaches; Insomnia; Itchy Nose; Mood changes; Red skin; Skin Rashes and Swollen Ankles. (Staying Healthy With Nutrition Elson M. Haas, M.D. 2006.).

The bowels and the lungs are the storage area of the body for everything that a person eats, drinks or breathes. However, the bowel storage system is based on a 16 hour day. Normal bowel movements should occur once daily as a minimum and three times maximum. Nevertheless two bowel movements would be ideal. The waste in your digestive system needs to be excreted in a timely manner to prevent it from being reabsorbed into the blood stream. (Page 744 and

747, Staying Healthy With Nutrition. Elsor M. Haas, M.D. Celestiae Arts, Berkeley, California 2006.)

Ridding the body of waste is known as detoxification. There are various methods to help your body to detox. The short term detox is through your daily diet, which as a suggestion could be:

1.) Radishes, which are natural detoxifiers
2.) Drink one small glass of salt water.
3.) Add spicy foods, hot peppers and cayenne pepper to your diet.
4.) Eats high fiber foods and olive oil.
5.) Drink lavender tea to detox the liver.
6.) Drink watermelon juice to detox kidney.
7.) Eat one tablespoon of raw unheated sauerkraut before each meal. Sauerkraut contains good bacteria for the digestive tract.
8.) Flaxseed and Bentonite clay (helps to bind metals for excretion).
9.) Eat Yogurt with each meal to obtain good digestive bacteria.
10.) Red grapes with seeds. Eat the grapes, but not the seeds throughout the day. Grapes with seeds are considered to be stronger in defending the immune system.
11.) Drink carrot juice for three consecutive days.
12.) Sweating causes pores in the skin to discharge toxins. A sauna or a steam room is most useful for this purpose.
13.) The supplement "reduced glutathione" and the herb milk thistle both detox the liver and chelates heavy metals.
14.) Drink a small portion of vinegar, if possible, apple cider vinegar, before each meal.

Also, longer detox periods include: Fasting on fruit juices and water for three consecutive days; a diet of steamed vegetables, fresh fruit and water for three consecutive days; store-bought cleanses; an old-fashioned enema works as well as any other method.

Fasting helps the body get rid of "acid wastes," which includes ammonia, a byproduct of protein metabolism.

Detoxification may be the key to avoiding cancer especially Breast Cancer. Toxins move through the body and if not removed through normal metabolism they are free to search out the fat, for toxins, becomes a safe haven. Once they become entrenched in the fat, a source of energy for the toxins, they begin to rapidly increase without interruption. Nonetheless, fat detoxification can only occur by burning off the fat either by exercise or diet. The detoxification process eliminates the toxins in the blood through excretion. Also, it is important to note that a woman's breast is mostly fat tissue, which is why detoxification is absolutely necessary.

Food plays an important function in providing nutrition to cells for proper metabolic activity. However, a lack of nutrients can have the opposite effect by affecting the way the genes are programmed.

Although your hereditary genes can predispose you to an inherited disease, it is not inevitable. Good nutrition may forestall or even prevent these predisposed genes from triggering a hereditary disease. Nonetheless, poor nutrition can cause the opposite effect by freeing the hereditary genes to wreak havoc on the body.

Children inherit genes from their parents; however, they also become recipients of their parents' eating habits. Bad eating habits on the part of parents may alter the DNA in the genes that are passed on to their children. The often used cliche, "you have good genes" is based on fact. Essentially, another well known cliche, "You are what you eat" is also based on fact; rather than myth.

CHAPTER THREE

Choosing a Multivitamin and Mineral Supplement

1) Look for high potency vitamins because diet alone cannot supply proper nutrition to the body. The soil no longer contains the abundance of vitamins and minerals that the land possessed seventy-five years ago when the animals fed upon the open range.

2) Look for high amounts of vitamins and minerals which are necessary to supply the interaction that is required for the body to manufacture enzymes and co-enzymes. Most vitamin supplements supply insufficient levels. Always look for the words “high potency” or the equivalent thereof on the label.

3) Look for vitamins designed separately for men and women since each has different needs.

For example, look for the following vitamins and their levels: Vitamin A (beta carotene)--5000 IU; Vitamin A (retinol) 2500 IU; Vitamin B1--75 mg; Vitamin B2--50mg; Vitamin B3–75mg; Vitamin B5--75mg; Vitamin B6--75mg; Vitamin C--500/1000 mg; Vitamin D--300 IU; Vitamin E--300 IU; Choline--100 mcg; Folic Acid--800 mcg and Biotin--400 mcg. Murray, M. (2006, February Ask Dr. Murray Newsletter, 1-2. The advantages of single dosages of herbal medicines). Also Vitamin B12--Taken as separate vitamins sublingual form (B12 cannot be absorbed once in the digestive tract)

MINERALS—Colloidal Minerals, also known as ionic minerals or trace minerals. Minerals should be taken in liquid form which allows for better absorption. These minerals do not have to be purchased separately. When you purchase Colloidal Minerals, the bottle includes each of the listed minerals.

Aluminum
Antimony
Arsenic
Barium
Beryllium
Bismuth
Boron
Bromine
Cadmium
Calcium
Cerium
Cesium
Chlorine
Chromium
Copper
Cobalt
Dysprosium
Erbium
Europium
Fluorine
Gadolinium
Gallium
Germanium
Gold
Hafnium
Holmium
Indium
Iodine
Iridium
Iron
Lanthanum
Lead
Lithium
Lutetium
Magnesium
Manganese
Molybdenum
Neodymium
Nickel
Niobium
Osmium
Phosphorus
Platinum
Polladium
Potassium
Praseodymium
Rhenium
Rhodium
Rubidium
Ruthenium
Samarium
Scandium
Selenium
Silicon
Silver
Sulfur
Sodium
Strontium
Tantalum
Tellurium
Terbium
Thallium
Thorium
Thulium
Tin
Titanium
Tungsten
Vanadium
Ytterbium
Yttrium
Zirconium
Zinc

CHAPTER FOUR

Telltale Warning Signs

Acne--Eliminate sugar from your diet and begin taking supplements--zinc; Omega 3; Vitamin A and Vitamin B complex.

Adult Acne–Take Niacinamide; Tea Tree Oil (apply topically)and Panothenic Acid cream (apply topically).

Arms (Skin tags under arms and on the back of the neck): Signs of Diabetes.

Arms (Chicken skin on arms)–Signifies a lack of sufficient essential fatty acids."

Blood pressure (High)--Insufficient Magnesium and Coenzyme Q10

Blood in the urine —May be an indication of a kidney problem.

Body (Yellow Body)--Low Thyroid or a liver problem.

Body Odor —Zinc deficiency and poor detoxification. See Chapter Two.

Body temperature (Low) accompanied by poor nails and hair--Low Thyroid.

Bruises (bruise easily)--Flavonoids and Vitamin K deficiency.--Easy Bruising – can be a sign of Leukemia, but can more likely be a sign of poor nutrition deficiency that if not corrected can lead to internal bleeding. Deficiencies may include the following: Vitamin K, flavonoids (keep blood vessels strong), dark fruits and vegetables. It will take 8 weeks or so to see a difference. Plus take Colloidal Minerals also known as Trace Ionic minerals (74 minerals). Also good multi-vitamin and a good herbal tea.

Energy – Rhodiola root enhances brain chemicals. It is available in capsule form.

Canker sores: Sign of poor stomach enzymes— Also connected to food allergies. It is recommended that you keep track of what you eat to try to determine which foods ignite the sores so they can be withdrawn from your diet. Another helpful item for canker sores is lactobacillus acidophilus, which aids in digestion. Also, when purchasing toothpaste, check the label to ensure it does not contain "sodium lauryl sulphate."

Chapped Lips—dehydration.

Colds (frequent)--Insufficient Vitamin C and zinc.

Cheeks (Rosy cheeks)–If you have rosy cheeks, it is a sign that your body contain sufficient iron; however, if the rosy cheeks are accompanied by rough dry skin or small bumps, it is a sign of Rosacea, which can also be detected due to a burning sensation in the cheeks. If the ailment is Rosacea, it is a sign of low stomach acid and low pepsin, which requires Hydrocloric Acid pills and Pepsin.

Feeling Cold–Always feeling cold could be a sign of anemia (Low iron), high blood pressure or poor circulation.

Complexion—A shiny reddish complexion signifies a person in good health, who has sufficient amounts of iron in the blood. In contrast, a lack of good complexion including pale lips indicates that there is a deficiency such as a lack of nutrients, vitamins, or poor diet.

Constipation--Caused by dehydration, low fiber diet; poor digestion and insufficient stomach acid (causes heartburn); add olive oil to meals and drink a small portion of vinegar, mixed with water, before each meal. Also, taking a double dose of milk of magnesia can help to end constipation.

Cravings (for sweets)—Insufficient Chromium, which is a mineral. This deficiency is extremely common among diabetics.

Ears--Cracked skin (behind ears)--Omega 3 and zinc.

Ears: Horizontal lines on ear lobes may indicate cardiovascular problems.

Ear lobes –Pink ear lobes (and a pink tongue) are a sign that there is sufficient iron in the blood.

Ears Ringing of—can be caused by over medication or excessive noise for prolonged periods of time. In conjunction, the origin of the problem could have a delayed reaction. For example, a person who listened to loud music (radio, stereo or modern day devices) may not feel the effects for years, but eventually, it can have a devastating effect on a person's hearing. The results are not always instant; however, it us strongly recommended that the volume of the device be at a moderate level. Organic garlic oil can be used to alleviate the ailment by using it as ear drops.

Eczema (Cracking of skin)--Omega 3, fatty acids and zinc deficiencies.

Eyes (Cloudy Eyes)--Cataracts—Signifies sugar problems. Excess sugar turns into cataracts.

Eyes (Dark Circles under the Eyes): signifies that a person requires more sleep. Nonetheless, sometimes, particularly with a child, the condition might be linked to something more serious.

Eyes (Horizontal creases on lower eye lids)--Allergies, hyperactivity—eliminate refined sugar and dairy products. Dark circles, along with horizontal creases on the lower eyelid are frequently associated with severe food allergies.

Eyes (dry eyes)--Insufficient Vitamin A and Omega 3.

Eyes (night blindness)--Insufficient Vitamin A and zinc.

Eyes (Red watery eyes)--Lack of Vitamin C.

Eyes (Puffy**)**-May be caused by a lack of proper sleep, poor digestion or even a food allergy.

Eyes (Vision Problems**)** It is important that you eat hefty portions of various fruits and vegetables, along with moderate consumption of meats. It is also helpful to take a high quality multi vitamin that contains Vitamin A, Vitamin D and calcium as recommended by the American Medicine Journal of Ophthalmology 1937. Also, when choosing your fruit, try to select dark fruit which are rich in flavonoids. Other helpful items to consider are the herb black currant and Hawthorne, both of which aid in the support of blood vessels.

Night blindness--eat hefty portions of spinach. Also, you can supplement with Vitamin A or raw carrots.

Eye health- The following supplements are helpful: glutathione an antioxidant; copper; lutein, contained in leafy green vegetables, is good for the health of the eyes; cysteine an amino acid, selenium; Vitamin E and Vitamin B-12. Also, to detox heavy metals take bentonite clay with water. The clay binds with the metals and escorts them to excretion.

Eyesight can also be fortified and improved by the following: broccoli, which contains sulphoraphane known to protect against UV damage. Also lutein and zeaxanthin (contained in broccoli, brussel sprouts, corn, egg yolks, honeydew melon, kale, lettuce) are good for the health of the eyes. Also, during World war II, pilots accidentally discovered that blueberries and bilberry (fruit) helped the rods in the eyes which improved their night vision.

Also, drink plenty of water to help detoxify the eyes. Apples, particularly the skin, are also excellent for detoxifying the eyes. Another fruit that is full of antioxidants (polyphenols) is red grapes (with seeds). Yet another natural supplement that is beneficial to the eyes is Colloidal Minerals.

Eye fatigue–it is extremely helpful for your eyes if you eat more carrots for beta carotine or you can get a more concentrated beta carotine, which is available in supplement form (ask for zeaxanthin). Many of you will remember the old saying about carrots being great for the eyes and on a personal note, once my eyesight seemed to be changing, a carrot-a-day was added to my diet and to my surprise, within about one week, the improvement in my eyesight became very noticeable. Since that time, the carrot has become a staple in my diet.

Your diet should include carrots, fruit and vegetables, along with supplements. During February 2006, the American Journal of Medicine Association produced a study that found an antioxidant filled diet was effective in preventing loss of vision. It was also discovered by the identical study that supplements were unable to produce similar results. A diet should include nuts, citrus fruits, fish and vegetables, such as broccoli and carrots. Other supplements that aid in maintaining good eyesight include Vitamins E and C, Beta Carotene, and Zinc, each of which will reduce the risk of macular degeneration while they work to strengthen eyesight.

Organic raw grapes contain phytochemicals that protect vision. Eat one handful daily or take a grape extract supplement. Other raw fruits and a vitamin supplement are helpful by producing antioxidants that combat free radicals.

Eat an apple a day and include the skin of the apple, which is the best part due to its content of fiber and because it contains pectin. Also, ginkgo biloba a free radical scavenger that also protects the eyes; take as directed. Other supplements include Vitamin E (take as directed); multi-vitamin; Colloidal Minerals (take as directed to obtain 67 trace minerals needed to sustain body functions).

Water- drink plenty of water to help keep the body detoxified through the process of urination which disposes toxins.

Broccoli has an antioxidant called sulphoraphane which helps to protect the eye from free radicals caused by UV light (ultra violet). Also, zinc, selenium, Vitamin A and digestive enzymes help to protect the eyes.

Other suggestions, known to be extremely helpful for the eyes includes: zinc; Vitamin C; eat large amounts of raw fruits including oranges, red grapes and strawberries. Also, Vitamin E supplement; Beta Carotene (the best source is raw carrots) which should be eaten on a daily basis. Sunflower seeds, pumpkin seeds and walnuts are also considered to be helpful for the health of the eyes. Celery is also good for the eyes. Eat some celery every day. Celery helps to improve the circulation of the blood and it also helps dilate blood vessels, including those of the eyes. By eating foods which are known to help protect the eyes, these same foods are helpful against macular degeneration, the major cause of blindness that affects the elderly.

Face (red scaly skin)--Insufficient Vitamin B-2 (riboflavin).
Fatigue--Could be a sign of Anemia—Vitamins; fruits; vegetables and meats are all sources of nutrition that fight fatigue. Fatigue can also be caused by a toxic body and if it is the cause, the liver needs to be detoxified. See Chapter Two on detoxification. Fatigue can also be caused by a lack of vitamin D. Sunlight is the best source for Vitamin D. It is important to be exposed to sunlight for about twenty minutes per day.

Exercise is also important and should be practiced on a daily basis. Exercise activates the pineal gland (it is also light activated),which releases melatonin and serotonin to regulate the cycles of a person's wakened hours and their sleep cycles. Do not wear sunglasses or block the light sensitive pineal gland. A quick source of energy can be acquired by taking the amino acid, tyrosine (capsule) combined with a magnesium (capsule). Remove the powder from the capsules then combine and mix in a small amount of water before drinking.
Feet—Numbness indicates poor circulation or the beginning stages of diabetes.
Fibrocystic disease- a common female problem, which is related to hormones. Daily use of high powered multi-vitamins that supply large doses of Vitamin A, Vitamin B-6, Vitamin C, Vitamin D and Vitamin E and zinc. Also, yet another valuable supplement is 74 minerals (Colloidal Minerals); take as directed. Eliminating chocolate, coffee and tea will usually improve the condition.
Fibromyalgia- is the combination of chronic pain, a lack of energy and weight gain. The cause is unknown. Some think it is caused by the body's reaction to stress. Take one drop of oregano oil (P-73) and mix in an herbal tea once a day. Continue the practice for two weeks. During the third week, drink the combination every third day. The mixture of the P-73 and an herbal tea works to detoxify the body.
Foot fungus -apply tea tree oil on the affected area or apply P-73

oregano oil, both of which are antifungal. Soaking the feet in salt water is also helpful.

Frequent urination- can be a vitamin or mineral deficiency, take B-complex, zinc, and magnesium. Can also be the beginning of prostate problems.

Forehead (Horizontal Wrinkles on forehead): Ulcers.

Gums--Bleeding gums are associated with periodontal disease. Often, this condition can be improved or corrected by using a folate mouthwash and by adding Coenzyme Q10 and folate to your diet.

Hair--for shiny healthy hair–apply two raw eggs to your hair ten minutes before you wash your hair.

Hair Dry– apply mayonnaise on your hair once a week and after waiting ten minutes, wash it out.

Hair Oily–after shampooing your hair, rinse with lemon juice.

Hair--The quality of the hair if poor, indicates a lack of healthiness.

Hair loss--Insufficient Biotin, Zinc and basic fatty acids may be causing hair loss. Thinning hair may be caused by poor digestion. Low stomach acids prevent proteins from being digested properly, which prevents the proteins from producing amino acids. Nails, as well as hair require amino acids. Also, low stomach acid causes poor mineral metabolism (low iron and low B-12. It is suggested that you take Betaine HCL (hydrocloric acid).

Hair loss may also be the result of a side effect of a pharmaceutical drug or chemotherapy. However, causes are not limited to those side effects. Other causes include:

Hair Premature gray--Insufficient B-12 and the mineral boron.

Hair Loss in Women–Whether the cause (of hair loss) is menopausal or not, you should use natural progesterone cream, which is available over the counter. Some women suffer from hair loss, which may be caused because of low amounts of iodine in the system. Low iodine may also cause depression and or weight gain.

→ **Malnutrition** can affect the hair and may be caused as a result of too much red meat or too much animal fat, which causes the scalp's pores to clog. Insufficient blood flowing to the scalp is another factor that can contribute to hair loss.

→ **Thyroid problems** (contribute to hair loss)- to do a self-test: for two days in the morning take your temperature under your armpit for 10 minutes. If your temperature is below 97.5 degrees you have a low thyroid. If your temperature is above 98.7 degrees you have an overactive thyroid. If you discover a problem, See also Thyroid Problems (page 167).

→ **Poor diet**, particularly an iron deficiency, which is not uncommon in women. The following foods are helpful: avocados; kale (high in iron); berries; dried fruits; whole grains; molasses; nuts; oats; olive oil; protein (fish, poultry, beans and nuts); sauerkraut (take 1tbsp before each meal to improve digestion and help to absorb nutrients; vegetables and seeds (pumpkin, sunflower, etc).

→ The following supplements are helpful: iron; zinc (take daily) along with copper; Biotin, which is found in brown rice is very good for the health of the hair. Biotin is also found in nuts, oats and brewers yeast; B Complex- take as directed. Other helpful supplements include: Vitamin C (helps to absorb the iron)–take daily or eat plenty of fruit; Vitamin E–(helps to keep the scalp healthy); fish oil and at least two cups of a multi-herbal tea daily. Other supplements that are helpful to the digestive system are HCL (hydrochloric acid tablets) and pancreatic enzymes. Take as directed on bottle.

→ Foods that you should not eat: white flour, white rice; white sugar, hydrogenated fats and processed foods. It is also important to eliminate milk from your diet because of the use of hormones and antibiotics that are given to cows to increase production may cause unintended effects on women who consume the milk.

Halitosis (bad breath)—can be caused by poor health, a sinus infection, a tooth infection or poor dental hygiene. The condition may be improved or corrected by using grapefruit seed extract or aloe as a mouth rinse. Mouth washes, which are known to help kill bacteria cannot distinguish between good bacteria and bad bacteria. Consequently, the use of grapefruit seed extract may be the better alternative because it does not affect the good bacteria. It also helps to reduce plaque.

Hands—Cold hands—If your hands remain cold in a warm environment, it may indicate poor circulation.

Hands Trembling—If your hands tremble, it may be caused from a lack of sufficient Magnesium and Vitamin B-1.

Hangovers--Vitamin B complex (all of the B Vitamins) helps to break down the alcohol. It is also recommended that you drink plenty of water to overcome dehydration, which is caused by the alcohol. You can also drink Gatorade which replenishes depleted electrolytes. Another remedy that reaches back to days of old is toast coated with honey. The toast and honey also works to replenish lost nutrients.

Headaches–take magnesium daily, which will help to reduce muscle tension, however, you should not use it if you suffer from a kidney problem. Magnesium is an essential mineral and about fifty percent of it is located in the bones. The remainder is primarily located in the body's organs and tissues. The blood contains only about one percent of magnesium, however, the body works tirelessly to maintain the blood levels of magnesium. If the kidneys are not fully functional, they are unable to excrete excess magnesium.

Heartburn --Low stomach acid—drink a small portion of Bragg's Apple Cider Vinegar, mixed with water before each meal or include a portion of vinegar on a salad.

Heel spurs–may be caused by a lack of calcium in the diet; however, it is also possible that the cause is from poor circulation. Another possible cause might be due to a lack of Vitamin K2 or Vitamin D; however, it could be due to a lack of minerals including the following: magnesium, copper, or boron.

Hemorrhoids–Use petroleum jelly and zinc oxide apply as needed. Use rutin also known as quercetin, an over the counter product. Use externally with liquid Vitamin C cream or oil, which will enhance the strength of the walls of the blood vessels. Also, a paste made of elm bark, jimson weed, pine tar, honey and yellow sulphur is also helpful. Apply it often. It is important that you consume plenty of water and olive oil to avoid constipation. Another remedy that is helpful is to insert ice cubes in the anal cavity to reduce the swelling of the hemorrhoids.

Herpes (HPV)–A virus that is difficult to combat; however, it is necessary to have a strong immune system. Supplements that can help to defeat the virus include selenium, colloidal trace minerals, glutathione, P73 oregano oil and amino acid lysine.

Hives--related to allergies and low stomach acid.

Hot flashes– may be caused by menopause. Take Vitamin B6 and oyster shell calcium as directed.

Immune system–A person's immune system can operate at maximum efficiency through the foods they consume. Herbs are an excellent way to provide the body with the necessary nutrients, including antioxidants vitamin minerals and enzymes to fight invading intruders. Herbs are also alkalizing to the body and keep our PH alkaline to fight viruses, bacteria, and yeast. Herbs essentially provide the cells with a protective shield. This shield is an oxygen rich body tissue that provides an unfriendly environment to these invading organisms. Part of this unfriendly environment is due to the plant kingdom inherent "electromagnetic vitality," which is the method by which the body's cells communicate with the cells of the brain.

Legs–If you detect brown or yellow coloring on the front of your legs, it may be an indication that there is a problem with insulin, which might be a sign of diabetes. Also, a condition known as Restless Leg Syndrome, which is caused by a toxic build-up in the legs' tissues can be helped by taking milk thistle and reduced glutathione.

Lips (Cracked Lips appearing in the corners of the mouth): Vitamin deficiency. Take Riboflavin, B-12 and B-complex.

Libido (Low libido in men**)--**Walnuts are very helpful. They are a good food that enhances sex drive.

Low cholesterol and low fat diets can lead to low sex drive. The body requires good fats, combined with the elimination of the following foods: fried foods; over processed foods; white vinegar and products that contain white flour products. Another cause of low sex drive could be poor circulation.

Muscle cramps–Cramps may indicate an insufficient amount of magnesium or potassium in the body.

Nails (Cracked Finger Nails)--Indicates a low level of stomach acid, a shortage of protein and of nutrients. The absence of sufficient amounts of proteins and nutrients being digested and absorbed into your body interferes with the natural growth of fingernails. However, it is also possible that the cause of cracks or chips on the fingernails can be attributed to a body's intolerance of refined sugar and in more severe cases, the root of the problem could be the thyroid. Fingernails naturally grow and or replace themselves rather quickly. The problem with nails, similarly to hair or skin, when not growing properly is easily detectable. Also, nails described as thin, weak or brittle can be associated with a low thyroid.

Nails (Black Splinters)–indicates anemia.

Nails (White spots on nails)--Indicates a zinc deficiency. Also, in some cases, white spots on the nails are an indication of gluten and or gliadin intolerance (Spru–celiac disease) or a deficiency in pancreatic enzymes.

Nails (spoon shaped)–indicates an iron deficiency.

Nose bleeds: High blood pressure.

Nose (Dermatitis on or "around" nose)–Take Vitamin B-6.

Roseacia –Usually noticeable in middle-aged people, especially women. Something triggers the rush of blood to the facial area which is the result of blood vessel dilation. People afflicted with Roseacia have difficulty caused by the blood vessels' failure to constrict which causes the blood vessels to stay dilated. The following items may be the cause that triggers the problem: alcohol; food allergies; hormone imbalance; nutrient deficiencies and poor digestion (most common cause).

Skin problems are usually one of the body's signals that something is wrong internally. The most common is poor digestion, usually associated with acid reflux as a side effect. This is a lack of stomach acid (hydrochloric acid) necessary for food digestion and a lack of good digestive system bacteria which aids in digestion and nutrient assimilation.

→ Take (HCL) hydrochloric acid tablets as directed.

→ Eat 1 tablespoon of raw unheated sauerkraut before each meal for good bacteria.

→ Eat yogurt often for good bacteria and take liquid acidophilus bifus, which has billions of good bacteria. Take before meals as directed.

→ Detoxify body – see Chapter Two on detox. Stored toxins end up in body tissue and try to exit the skin. Also due to poor digestion.

→ Drink a multi-herbal tea for nutrients and detoxification.

→ Take a high potency multivitamin.

→ B-complex –Take as directed.

→ Take Vitamin B-12 sublingual– take daily.

→ Milk thistle capsules – an herb that protects the liver and aids in detoxification –take daily as directed.

→ Drink lots of water to help detoxifation.

→ Eat lots of fiber to aid detox. Fiber also carries off excess cholesterol and toxins.

→ Hormone imbalance. Low progesterone or birth control pills maybe the culprit. If you use hormone replacement make sure they are not synthetic.

Skin (Dry)–Usually due to the lack of essential fatty acids. Take lots of Vitamin A as directed. Also cut back on foods such as coffee, eggs, meat, milk and vinegar, which causes the blood to be acidic. Take Colloidal Minerals and a multi vitamin plus flaxseed Also, take digestive enzymes for nutrient absorption. If you have dry skin, use liquid Vitamin C and grape seed extract mixed together (apply topically). To eliminate toxins, you should detox and take Fish oil (Omega 3), zinc, selenium, Vitamins A, B complex, D and E are helpful. You can also apply unrefined wheat germ oil, which acts as a moisturizer for the skin.

Skin Cancer-–Make a paste by mixing Vitamin E mixed with DMSO (available at health food stores) and apply topically two times daily. Curaderm a product, made from eggplant, and sold in health food stores may also be helpful. Dried oregano is an anti-cancer herb that should be eaten with meals. It may cause the cancerous cells to dry up and flake off.

Skin problem--wash skin with vinegar and eat lemons. Combine the lemons and vinegar with a daily cup of herbal tea with one drop of lavender added. Take for two weeks for liver detoxification. Afterward, add one drop of lavender every 3rd day for maintenance. You can also detox with reduced glutathione or lemon water.

Skin problems may be the result of a thyroid disorder. Kelp and tea support thyroid. Bentonite clay, used in conjunction with detoxification works to kill bacteria and pathogens. The bacteria and pathogens can develop resistance to antibiotics; however, they are vulnerable to the clay. You can also use Yucca powder to bind harmful fats and toxins and pass them to excretion. Also, if you are stung by a bee, by placing a penny on the spot of the sting, the penny acts as an antiseptic.

Smell (reduced sense of)–Insufficient zinc.

Taste (reduced sense of)–Insufficient zinc.

Teeth (loose)–Brush your teeth with a combination of baking soda

and hydrogen peroxide (food type) and rinse with salt water.
Thyroid swelling–Indicates a possible lack of iodine.
Tongue (Geographic Tongue--raised grooves and contour): Vitamin deficiency.

Requires folate, zinc and B-12, all of which are contained in leafy green vegetables. ⇛Another source for folate and B-12, chlorella, can be acquired at natural food stores.
Tongue (Pale Tongue)--Anemia–Requires eating additional fruit and adding additional iron in your daily diet. Also, it is possible that the anemia is caused by gastrointestinal bleeding; you should check your stool.
Tongue (Rosy Red Tongue)--You are healthy. The sign of good health.
Tongue (Swollen and Scalloped Tongue):

Related to food allergies.
Urine–Foamy Urine–Excess sugar. Check for diabetes.
Varicose veins: To reduce swelling it is suggested that you try a product called Arnica which is made from the comfrey plant.
Poor circulation in the legs causes the blood to pool. The blood vessels need to be strengthened by taking trace minerals, flavonoids (dark fruit and vegetables) and a good herbal tea that includes Ginkgo Biloba, horse chestnut and bilberry. Also Vitamin E, magnesium and a high fiber diet decreases pressure in the abdomen, which allows better circulation of the blood moving from the legs back to the heart. Poor circulation and veins that lose their elasticity need the herbs Gotu Kola, ginkgo biloba, niacin, raw garlic and Vitamin E.

CHAPTER FIVE

Did You Know?

Acids (Essential Fatty Acids Omega 3)--Children should take EFA (Essential Fatty Acids – Omega 3), which is good for the growth of the brain. They also contain prostaglandins which fight infection.

Age related deficiencies--include the lack of vitamins, including B12, minerals, and fatty acids. Due to poor digestion, enzyme output by the stomach, intestines and pancreas (bile) is reduced as a person ages. Another cause of poor indigestion is the lack of raw fruit and vegetables in the diet. Over-cooking food destroys the enzymes and trace minerals. The digestive system needs probotics, yogurt, sauerkraut and more raw foods for it to function properly. Digestive enzymes also help with arthritis, asthma, irritable bowels and colitis. The digestive enzymes are especially important for people suffering from ill-health or those people who are recovering from a health problem.

Calcium channel blockers--For those people who take calcium channel blockers, the blockers are designed to keep calcium outside of the arteries where it relaxes them; rather than inside where the calcium hardens and tightens the arteries. The side effects include fatigue, headaches, swollen ankles, constipation and heart failure. Calcium channel blockers also effect the muscles; however, with fewer side effects. (The Informed Consumers Pharmacy, Ellen Brown and Lynne Paige Walker (Doctors of Pharmacy) Page 62 Carroll and Graf Publications. N.Y. 1990).

High Blood Pressure (HBP) can be the result of the kidneys retaining too much fluid, which may be caused from excessive salt. The salt makes the blood more dense. Consequently, the heart has to work too hard, particularly if the arteries are constricted. Taking Ace inhibitors blocks the angiotensin enzymes which stop the blood vessels from constricting. Side effects include coughing, rashes and the loss of potassium and coenzyme. The loss of potassium is easily spotted because the urine turns into a deep yellow color. Potassium and Coenzyme Q10 are both necessary to keep the heart functioning.

Corticosteroids–some drugs that treat asthma should only be used for acute attacks. Corticosteroids, manufactured by drug companies, replace natural steroids produced by adrenal glands to reduce inflamation and open airways in the chest. However, corticosteroids prevent the body's natural reaction to allergens and stop the adrenals from producing natural hormones. Side effects from using corticosteroids, include bone loss, easy bruising and gaining weight. Also, when corticosteroids are prescribed for children, side effects can include emotional problems and possibly growth problems.

Complex carbohydrates--lower cholesterol. Whole grains and barley may block the production of cholesterol in the liver. Also, soluble fiber helps transport excess cholesterol out of the body: soluble fiber includes food such as; oats, bran muffins and oat bran cereal and other complex carbohydrates including those contained in chile, peas, black eyed peas, sweet potatoes, bananas, oranges, corn, charred beans, rye bread, whole wheat bread, broccoli, kidney beans, navy beans, cauliflower, zucchini and whole grain bread.

Another soluble fiber, oats, produces a gel-like substance that reduces cholesterol absorption. Refined foods lack sufficient fiber and consequently, the deficiency prevents the consumption of refined food to satisfy hunger.

Counting Calories, A Solution To The Diet

→ Increase complex carbohydrates.
→ Increase the daily amount of water you drink.
→ Increase fiber intake.
→ Reduce fat (high fat equals high calories).
→ Reduce sugar and salt.

Sodium--The body requires a fluid to salt ratio, which is monitored by the kidneys to maintain balance. Sodium holds more fluid, which increases the density of blood. Consequently, excessive sodium taxes the heart by making it work harder to pump the blood. Also, sodium causes blood vessels to constrict, which can cause further complications, specifically high blood pressure.

Olive oil--reduces low density lipoproteins (LDL) and it raises high density lipoproteins (HDL). Italians and Greeks consume large amounts of olive oil and that is why they have low heart attack rates. Also, it is important to know that although your total cholesterol count may climb due to the consumption of olive oil, the LDL will not climb; rather, it will be decreased. Therefore, even if a person's cholesterol increases, as long as the LDL count remains low, the total cholesterol count has no adverse impact on the health of the arteries. It is important that you remember not to heat olive oil higher than 350 degrees or it will damage the original chemical consistency.

Gene Control –You have heard how our DNA chromosomes dictate our body characteristics, but they also control how our body reacts to nutrients or even no nutrients (toxins). That's why everything we eat, drink or breathe the body's metabolism knows what to do with it or without it. The study or nutrients impact on the body's ability to communicate cell to cell (transcription factors) is called nutrigenomics. Consequently you are what you eat has been partly laid out for you by your heredity (DNA). So if someone says "you have good genes," it's truer than you think.

Enzymes--The more enzymes in your stomach, the healthier you will be. Enzymes are protein molecules that create a chemical reaction, but without causing harm to the enzymes. They are comprised of proteins, minerals and white blood cells that attack invaders (bad bacteria and viruses). By eating more raw food, you will increase the amount of enzymes in your body, particularly in your pancreas. Cooking destroys enzymes. A book, "*The Enzymes Treatment of*

Cancer and its Scientific Basis." published during 1907 by John Berad, PHD, an embryologist, wrote that "Cooked food takes much longer to digest and it may irritate the lining of the entire intestinal tract. It could also lead to leaky gut syndrome, which occurs when undigested foods enter the blood stream and become free radicals."

Raw foods, however, contain the necessary enzymes which allows the raw food to rot. When your food is cooked, these necessary enzymes (free radical fighters) are destroyed and prevented from entering your system where they would otherwise join in the task of building your immune system. In conjunction, it is imperative that the body contains large numbers of free radical fighters to ensure that the body's immune system is functioning properly. Enzymes are shuttled through the body by proteins; consequently, the lack of proteins causes a lack of enzymes. Vegetarians should be aware of potential B-12 deficiency because meat is the only source of B-12.

The upper part of the stomach is the area of pre-digestion. Live foods are predigested in their own enzymes, including saliva glands. Nevertheless, an over abundance of cooked food in the digestive tract requires the body's immune system and pancreas to provide enzymes that help to digest the enzyme-depleted cooked foods. However, if the pancreas is too often called upon to produce enzymes, the pancreas will become enlarged, similarly to an athlete who often has an enlarged heart. The more cooked food you eat the faster you age because the body has to work much harder to metabolize the food.

Sixty-four enzymes exist to help the body repair itself and to get rid of waste. Cooked food, however, sidesteps this process. Some people who suffer from Leukemia go into remission when cooked food is eliminated from their diet. Eating raw foods never causes a person to get fat. Also, grilled meat contains a large number of toxins including heterocyclic amines (HCA) which are cancer causing compounds. Spices, which contain antioxidants help to reduce HCA.

Examples of typical total cholesterol counts in various parts of the world are:
United States–The average count is 215-300; Asia-130-180; Latin America–125-140; Mediterranean–140-180 and Third World–100-140.

Statins can alter liver function by interfering with the metabolism of cholesterol. Side effects of statins include liver damage and heart damage. One solution to cholesterol problems (high cholesterol) is diet, rather than a prescribed pill. The proper diet includes more soluble fiber from fruits and vegetables, beans and grain. Soluble fiber binds with excess cholesterol and carries the cholesterol to excretion.

You should also reduce your sugar intake because when sugar intake is excessive, it becomes a triglyceride. Also, it is important to reduce your consumption of saturated fat; however, some saturated fat from meat is good and also from dairy products. Most importantly, trans-fats which are found in fried food and processed food should be avoided.

Your diet should include olive oil, which brings down the LDL's and the antioxidants; turmeric (herb); cayenne pepper (increases metabolism); green or herbal tea. The tea works to stabilize blood sugar and it also has cardiovascular benefits. Tea also strengthens teeth and acts as a detergent that dissolves fats.

Other foods that should be included in your diet are: red grapes, red wine, cherries, cranberries, artichokes; leafy green vegetables and fruit. Bitter herbs may cause the liver to activate the gall bladder, which then produces more bile, which lowers cholesterol and starts the peristalis (muscle contractions in intestines) to keep waste moving through the body's digestive tract on its natural course. It also prevents the cholesterol from remaining in the intestines and the colon to be reabsorbed back into the blood.

Tanning Salons--The particular type of lighting, (U.V–ultra violet) is known to stimulate a person's blood flow and produce new skin tissue, known as collagen, which is a connective tissue that holds the cells together. The ultra violet lighting gives off wave lengths for blood flow and Vitamin D.

Skin cells, which are exposed to ultra violet radiation, create brown pigment. The pigment in turn forms a shield, which protects the cells from additional exposure to the UV rays by darkening the skin, more commonly known as tanning. UV radiation is produced by the sun, but also by artificial means such as a tanning salon or a tanning bed. Nevertheless, some studies show that excessive exposure to UV radiation is harmful to a person's health. Other studies strongly urge people to avoid tanning salons to lessen the possibility of getting skin cancer.

Splenda is produced in a laboratory; however, it is marketed as a natural product. Splenda metabolizes into a non-sugar called sucralose, which modifies intestinal bacteria by changing the PH and weakening the body's ability to absorb nutrients.

Low Libido (or E D as it is known) can sometimes be easily corrected (See also Chapter Six pg #178). Just follow a detoxification with a diet of organic fruits, vegetables, wild fish and free range meats. Avoid processed foods, which contain lots of preservatives and chemicals. Also, refrain from using white sugar and products that contain white flour. Another food product that should be avoided is fried foods (contains bad fats).

Vitamin K which is manufactured in your intestines helps to prevent calcification of the arteries. It is important to have good digestion and good bacteria in the intestines. Pharmaceutical drugs and antibiotics sometimes kill good bacteria and simultaneously they can prevent Vitamin K from being created.

Sugar plus proteins (amino acids), otherwise known as glycation, makes the arteries hard and less flexible, which can cause high blood pressure, cataracts, cardiovascular disease, erectile dysfunction and diabetes. The first parts of the body to suffer are the areas within the smallest blood vessels which are contained in the brain and the testicles. The poison from Insect sprays are now a common ingredient found in fruits and vegetables. If they are not released by the liver through detoxification, they can settle in the body's tissues. If so, the need for further detoxification or fasting becomes necessary.

Fasting has been a custom in many religions for centuries. And the custom has also been handed down through the ages by various ethnic cultures, based upon the belief that fasting is healthy. By fasting, the body is compelled to metabolize fat from the body's tissues, which releases the toxins to the blood and liver for detoxification and afterward excretion. See also, Diet, page 111.

→ **Yams**–Yams are a fine source of fiber and they also help to purify the kidneys and the spleen.

→**Poor PH** –is an acidic environment for muscle problems, heart disease, diabetes, influenza and a variety of diseases including cancer.

→**Calcium supplements** –The best source to take for absorption is calcium carbonate, but keep in mind that an individual needs Vitamin D, magnesium, copper, strontium, and boron for maximum absorption, which helps to keep the calcium liquid in the blood. The supplements also aid in the prevention of hardening of the arteries, kidney stones or calcified joints (which may be mistaken for arthritis.

Silica–stored in hair and skin–good for tinnitus, acne pimples, cracked nails, psoriasis, nervous system support and bone strength.

Raw honey, usually white in color, is a very good source of enzymes, vitamins and minerals. Do not overheat heat the honey, because with some honey, the heating (pasturization) will kill the enzymes. Also, raw honey mixed with the herb thyme, produces thymol, which is good for a sore throat and for colds. Also, raw honey helps to detoxify the body and it is anti-inflammatory.

Ginger–good for digestion. Ginger also fights colds and mild inflammatory problems.

Phosphoric Acid, which is contained in carbonated soda, depletes the calcium in a person's bones.

Potassium(contained in bananas and figs)--lowers blood pressure. Potassium is also helpful against muscle cramps.

Garlic–Garlic, which contains eighty sulphur compounds, helps to kill viruses and bacteria.

Cayenne pepper–Cayenne pepper mixed with water is a good mixture to drink if a person is suffering from a heart attack. The combination of the pepper and water is an identical substitute for nitroglycerine.

Lemons–Lemons enhance antioxidants and the absorption of nutrients. They also aid in detoxification. Eating lemons on a daily basis is a healthy habit.

Cholesterol medicine–May give you dry skin because it depletes the fat in the tissue and the skin requires cholesterol to keep the skin elastic and soft.

Popcorn–Popcorn (excluding popcorn suitable for the microwave) is high in fibre and antioxidants, for fighting free radicals (cells that are out of control). Also. popcorn is low in fat and high in fiber.

Vitamin D–helps detox the mercury that can accumulate in the brain of those people who consume large amounts of fish including fresh water and ocean species. Vitamin D also assists in the detoxification of body tissues by increasing glutathione production. It also helps eliminate bile acids, a byproduct of digestion. Vitamin D also plays an important part in fighting depression and it aids in the good health of the bones.

Yarrow–yarrow lowers blood pressure and dilates blood vessels.

DMSO (dimethylsulfoxide) –A byproduct of garlic oil is a free radical scavenger and it is anti-inflammatory.

Turmeric–a yellow herb from India that penetrates the membranes of cells to strengthen their effectiveness.

Parsnips–Contains Vitamin C, Potassium, phosphorus which aids in the fight against skin disorders, including acne.

Avocado–contains Vitamin E, Potassium monounsaturated fat (nature's butter) folate, fiber and lutein. The lutein in the avocado protects against hardening of the arteries. Lutein also helps to protect the eyes from getting cataracts and macular degeneration.

Pomagranates–contain fiber, Vitamin C, and potassium. Pomagranates also reduce plaque in the arteries and they contain many antioxidants that fight off disease.

Bananas–help to lower cholesterol and relieve heartburn. They contain fibre and potassium and they also help to calm an upset stomach.

Apples (with skin)–help to lower cholesterol and they decrease the risk of lung cancer.

Parsley –is good for the control of cholesterol, depression, PMS, and it also strengthens kidneys and it is a diuretic. Parsley is also very helpful in eliminating bad breath.

Oats–are complex carbohydrates that the cells use for energy. Oats are also a source of protein and they help control high blood pressure. In addition, oats are good for the gall bladder and the liver.

Garlic– keeps the body's chemistry balanced and it also acts as a blood purifier. Garlic is also instrumental in reducing artery plaque. Garlic also contains 80 separate sulphur compounds that help to improve the immune system.

Tomatoes–cherry tomatoes are more nutritional and the skin is the most nutritional part of the tomato.

Almonds-a good source of magnesium.

Cilantro–is a natural metal chelate (detoxification) for mercury. People who consume a large amount of fish in their diet become susceptible to ingesting mercury at high levels.

Vegetables–contain enzymes although the more you heat vegetables the more enzymes you lose. Raw vegetables are better. Enzymes help in detoxification and they are the catalyst that place the immune system into high gear.

Energy–B-12--supplements are available at health stores that should be taken sublingually, (under the tongue) to increase energy. Meat products contain B-12, which is stored by the body for prolonged periods of time. B-12 deficiencies are rare; however, the deficiency is common in vegetarians.

Sugar substitutes–cause the pancreas to begin pumping insulin out of the pancreas instantly as the sweetness is sensed by the tongue; however, not being sugar, there is none (sugar) to be transferred to the cells. This leads to insulin in the blood getting trapped, causing the body to crave more sugar. Also, excess insulin may lead to unwanted weight gain, fluid retention and it accelerates the aging process.

Moles–The herb blood root made into a paste may help eradicate.

Cosmetics–may be full of toxins, impurities, endocrine disruptors, estrogens and other irritants. Be cautious when selecting your cosmetics.

Pre-surgery herbs: Ginkgo Biloba; Grape seed extract and Milk thistle.

Echinacea–taken daily can lessen the risk of infection

Gotukola–an herb that strengthens the veins and the capillaries

Dandruff–After shampooing your hair, rinse with white vinegar.

Apples–good for asthma and a source of good fibre. Apples also increase the level of acetylcholine, a neurotransmitter (nerve signals) and they help to protect the body from free radicals.

Grape seed extract –acts as an excellent killer of germs if you suffer from a cold or the flu.

Oregano oil–for hiccups, coughs, eczema, psoriasis, athlete's feet, earache, canker sores, cold sores and diarrhea.

Sauerkraut and Yogurt–Each contains common stomach bacteria that is necessary for good digestion.

Niacin–lowers pulse and opens blood vessels.

Asthma–Magnesium relaxes airways.
Cod liver oil–an old time supplement for Vitamin D and Omega 3. Cod liver oil also relieves constipation and helps to relive arthritis pain.
Selenium-a mineral and antioxidant contained in canned tuna, garlic and turkey. It protects cells against sun damage and it helps to protect the prostate.
Beta Carotene–antioxidant contained in sweet potatoes and carrots and it protects the skin from sun burn. It also helps metabolize estrogen.
Chicken–high in Vitamin B-3, which dilates blood vessels and helps to keep blood pressure down.
Lead in some lipstick www.cosmeticdatabase.com
Bone broth soup--good for arthritis and it helps to rebuild cartilage.
Bonemeal–which contains two trace minerals (Boron and strontium) acts as a cement which hardens the bones.
SAM-e–A naturally occurring amino acid that is manufactured by the body, however in some people, not enough is produced. Take as directed. SAM-e also enhances a person's memory.
Blueberry leaf–keeps blood sugars stable and alpha Lipoic acid will absorb excessive sugar.
Acid Base Balance-

PH is like a swimming pool; if the PH is too low, the water turns cloudy. Acidic water can rot the pipes. That is why the pipes used in pools are pvc, which are immune to acid. However, your body is not immune. The body sometimes can be harshly affected, including cell degeneration in the form of cancer, Parkinson's disease, organ failure, fatigue, constant colds and a number of other ailments including weight gain associated with antigens (viruses and bacteria).

The body was designed to be alkaline but over-farming the land has caused a loss of nutrients in our food supply. Other examples of modern-day farming techniques that affect our health include the way that animals (raised for food) are fed. Animals originally grazed on free range, however, at present, many animals are grain fed and their feed is supplemented by antibiotics and hormones.

Farming in a general sense has changed drastically. We are a world away from the fresh unsprayed vegetables and fruit that were grown on the farms that were active 100 years ago. Even the grass feed of the animals of yesteryear is now subjected to chemical sprays.

PH is also kept in balance with the lungs when they exhale acidic toxins. Urine, feces and sweat also release acidic acid and toxins. However, an overload of acidic acid and toxins eventually ends up in body tissue where the positive charged cells interfere with the other cells normal function. Conversely, an alkaline body with negative charged cells bonds with other cells to enhance their normal function. For example, acidic PH is an environment that inhibits nutrients assimilation and increases the oxidative cycle by using up blood oxygen where bacteria and viruses thrive. Lack of oxygen also affects our energy level.

Baker's Yeast–helps to remove bad bacteria and viruses. A substitute for Baker's Yeast, which is available over the counter is Eipcor.

Bee pollen–contains enzymes that are beneficial to the lungs.

Curing disease through oxygen rich blood

Oxygen filled blood helps keep you alkaline and wards off disease like cancer, but if you have cancer, trying to achieve an oxygen rich alkaline blood should be your goal. This goal can only be achieved through diet which means no meat, soda, sugar or processed foods. Instead, a diet consisting of free range poultry, raw vegetables, raw fruit, onions and garlic is desirable. Onions and garlic, which contain sulfuric compounds are especially helpful. However, sulfuric compounds, much like vitamins A, D, E and K, need an oil to aid in absorption. For instance, flaxseed oil or fish oil can be ,added to the diet. Also, a calcium supplement that contains Vitamin D and magnesium is a valuable source of stimulation for the production of oxygen.

Grapeseed extract–a derivative of whole grape seeds. The extract is a bioflavonoid that contains an abundance of Vitamin E and is known to increase the strength of blood vessels, while also helping to protect them.

Dental Hygiene–Bad bacteria in the mouth can sometimes cause problems other than tooth decay. Frequent brushing helps to eliminate bad bacteria. Also, Flossing lowers C-reaction protein in the blood. If you use a mouthwash, select one that does not contain alcohol, which kills good bacteria along with bad bacteria and by destroying the good bacteria, it increases the chances of tooth decay.

Artificial Flavorings–Artificial flavorings, created through chemistry; rather than natural sources, contain foreign substances, which can cause side effects.

Hot Tubs–If you use a hot tub, it is paramount that the water is sanitized by chlorine or a similar product to prevent infections caused by folic hair bacteria (pseudomonas).

Eye Twitches –Can be caused by excessive amounts of caffeine, chocolate, or pills.

Appendix–The appendix is an integral component of the lymph system, which are glands of white blood cells that eliminate unwanted bacteria, viruses and other pathogens. The appendix, once thought of as having no important body function is now considered as a very significant part of the body function (detoxification) and should not be removed unless it becomes absolutely necessary.

Leafy Green Vegetables–They contain chlorophyl, which helps the body to restore cells and absorb minerals. Leafy green vegetables also work to keep your PH up to satisfactory levels.

Fat–The consumption of good fats aids the skin's elasticity. The fats also help to produce oil, which builds a barrier that protects the body from bad bacteria.

Fat Cells–Fat cells are a source of C-reactive protein, which when accumulated in high amounts may indicate a potential heart problem. Fat cells also work to reduce the hormone leptin, which controls hunger and satisfaction signals. However, all fat cells are not destructive; rather, the body also contains good fat cells that work to assist the body to absorb nutrients. They also store and distribute vitamins. In conjunction, good fat is contained in meat, the sole source of Vitamin B-12. Despite the myth that meat is bad for human consumption, it is a fact that many cultures that have heavy meat consumption, the people are considered to be very healthy, primarily because they eat range-fed meat and poultry.

Quinoa–Quinoa, not a widely known food is a amino acid-rich (protein) seed that is often used as a substitute for potatoes and pasta. Quinoa is gluten free. It is also low in sugar content, while it is high in fiber, magnesium, potassium and protein.

Water consumption–The body requires large amounts of water. Drinking water with lemon added helps keeps the kidneys alkaline and it can help to prevent kidney stones.

Raw Carrots–Raw carrots are a fine source of Vitamin A and they act as free radical scavengers which attack and devour mutated cells, essentially eliminating free radical cells that otherwise would cause damage to the body. Raw carrots also help to keep the skin moist. In addition, raw carrots as stories related through the ages, are genuinely excellent for the eyes.

Cooking Oils–When cooking at temperatures above 350 degrees, use saturated fat, cocoanut oil, butter or lard. When cooking at temperatures under 300 degrees, use avocado oil, macadamia or olive oil.

Sea Salt–Sea salt, which contains trace minerals including iodine is good for the thyroid; however, salt contains only a small amount of iodine. Normally, you will need to acquire iodine from additional sources.

Vitamin E–The best source for Vitamin E is alpha tocopherol.
Vitamin K –Vitamin A is created by good bacteria in the intestines.
Magnesium–Magnesium produces a hormone (calcitonin) that helps to keep calcium from entering soft tissue, while it diverts calcium to the bones.
Sauna–The use of a sauna is good for detoxification because it causes the body to sweat profusely and in so doing, helps the body to expel toxins. Using a sauna is also good for anyone suffering from diabetes because it lowers blood sugar, which simultaneously lowers insulin usage.
Hangovers–Eating honey and toast before drinking will help to reduce the lingering effects of a hangover. The combination works to clear the alcohol from the blood.
Alcohol Craving–Craving alcohol is usually caused by a mineral deficiency.
Spine (Alignment)–It is possible to give yourself a quick test to determine whether or not your spine is aligned. Move your head from left to right and then from right to left. If there is no restriction during the movement, it indicates that the spine is correctly aligned.
However, if you sustain some difficulty, you spine is probably out of alignment. If the latter occurs, you should see a chiropractor for examination or treatment.
Meat Gristle–Meat gristle, fat and bone marrow is the same as chondroitin, a molecule found in cartilage. The gristle aids in the repair of cartilage.
Washing the body too often removes the body's protective bacteria barrier – plus coating the skin with moisturizers and powder to take the place of your natural oils is harmful. Look at the ingredients of the products you put on your skin and anything not natural is also absorbed into your blood stream.

Clean your arteries–make a cocktail of Vitamins C, E and D, inositol, hexaniacinate (a form of Vitamin B-3), L-carnitine, liver oil and a multi vitamin. Also, take lecithin, celery and garlic.

Plastic Surgery– If you're considering plastic surgery on your face, make sure you see a dermatologist to examine any spots on your face for cancer. The reason I suggest this is a client of mine contacted three plastic surgeons for cosmetic work on her face. After seeing two of the plastic surgeons she mentioned to the third surgeon that she was concerned about the three brown spots on her face. His response was to see a dermatologist since he had no idea what they were. The visit to the dermatologist proved the spots to be cancerous and one of the spots was near her eye. They were subsequently removed.

The point I'm making is that the plastic surgeons showed no concern about the spots and if the woman had gone ahead with the surgery without consulting with a dermatologist, the spots, despite being cancerous, would have been concealed and still deadly. In addition, the cancer would have continued to spread without being detected.

Prostate health –avoid artificial fat for example potato chips or the artificial fat called olestra. Increase the amount of carotenoids like lycopenes. That helps protect the prostate from cancer.

Egg Yolk--supplies lecithin to the body to prevent cholesterol absorption. Egg yolk is also a fat used in non-stick sprays for cooking, Egg yolk also stops cholesterol from sticking to the arteries, which lowers the risk of clogged arteries. Egg yolk also aids in the protective myelin sheath that forms around nerve linings. However, if you don't eat egg yolk your body still produces lecithin, but not enough to guarantee good health. Also, lecithin is the ingredient used in non-stick sprays (cooking).

Chemotherapy--A side effect of Chemotherapy is that the saliva glands stop working, which will lead to the loss of your teeth.

Women--Too much sleep–Women (ages 50-79) who get more than 9 hours sleep are more likely to have a stroke than those getting 6 hours or fewer, according to a study conducted by the University of North Carolina School of Public Health.

MSG–A chemical formula that causes excessive heart palpitations, asthma, and ADHD. It is also known to kill brain cells. MSG is also known by several other names, including "hydrolyzed vegetable protein.

Soy—may be associated with many problems, including various cancers (including breast cancer) and thyroid problems. Soy can imitate estrogen and it may reduce absorption of calcium. Copper, iron, magnesium and zinc.

Cod liver oil – an old time remedy used by many health specialists when treating depression, heart disease, high blood pressure and rheumatoid arthritis. Cod liver oil contains Omega 3. You should also take Vitamin D3, in conjunction with the Omega 3.

Poor circulation test – use a tourniquet around the arm to block the blood flow or use a blood pressure testing cuff with the blood not flowing wait until the index finger on the same hand starts to get cold then loosen the cuff or tourniquet and see how long it takes for blood to circulate back to the finger. The longer it takes the worse you circulation.

Fish oil--helps to transport a hormone called leptin to the brain to signal that you are full. Fish oil also reduces triglycerides and it reduces the risk of getting rheumatoid arthritis.

Trans fats-- includes vegetable oil, shortening, and anything that states on the label that it is hydrogenated or partially hydrogenated.

Scented candles – many contain formaldehyde and other ingredients which can produce headaches and allergic reactions.

Horse Radish--contains calcium, iron, magnesium, phosphorus and Vitamin C. It is also good for circulation and a detoxification.

However, you should avoid horse radish if you have an under active thyroid.

Aging – the goal is to eliminate oxidation. Oxidation is the byproduct of cellular activity when exposed to oxygen. The ensuing byproducts are in themselves damaging toxins that must be extracted from the body. Glutathione plays a major role in detox. Detoxification of toxic compounds. The body makes glutathione but as we get older our production levels of this detoxifier decreases.

Aging is a natural process; however, it is accelerated when protein is metabolized and oxidized which transforms the proteins into toxins. The failure to detoxify and remove the metabolized proteins that have oxidized permit them to accumulate as toxins.

Suggested supplements:

→**Multivitamins**

→**L-arginine–dilates blood vessels.**

→**Colloidal Minerals** – 74 trace minerals.

→**Fish oil**

→**Reduced glutathione**–helps to detox the cells.

Manganese–helps to build strong cell membranes called collagen. The word Manganese is taken from the Greek word magic.

→**Milk Thistle**-–helps to protect and detox the liver.

→**Multi Herbal Tea** -–contains antioxidants and enzymes. The tea also aids in detoxification.

→**Liquid oxygen**--Good for cell energy, detoxification and it enhances the immune system. The product is available over the counter. Take as directed.

→**Liquid Vitamin D3**–During the winter season most people have a Vitamin D3 deficiency.

→**CoQ10** –artery health – take as directed.

→**Max 3**–An over the counter product that contains Maitake mushrooms and the herb, cats claw. Take as directed.

→**Epi Quercian** –An over the counter product that contains amino acids, lysine and minerals. Take as directed.

→**Wormwood** – A herb known for its anti-cancer compounds. Take as directed.

Pancreas Health–Take the pancreatic enzymes, Trypsin and Chymotrypsin. Also take Vitamin B-12 (available in capsule form and in nasal spray. Vitamin B-12 in its natural form is contained in red meat, poultry and yeast.

Tomatoes--contain lycopene, which helps to reduce cholesterol. Cooking the tomato increases the lycopene content.

Chocolate--contrary to popular belief, is not helpful to the aging process if it is commercial chocolate. Cocoa, however, without sugar has benefits that contain 300 compounds protein, fat, iron, zinc, copper, calcium, fiber. Cocoa is also beneficial for bone strength and for nail strength, due to sulfur compounds contained in cocoa. Cocoa also raises the pulse rate and it activates the adrenal glands to produce relaxing hormones. Commercial chocolate is known to prevent the absorption of vital minerals due to its oxalic acid content. The oxalic acid is corrosive to tissue and it binds to metals, which causes the kidneys and stomach to become irritated.

LDL--Your LDL count should be no lower than 100 for good cardiovascular health – LDL's are necessary for the transportation of cholesterol.

Gallbladder contractions are a function of the digestive process when eating fatty meals. However, if a stone exists, the contraction puts pressure on it and causes pain. If the stone blocks the bile duct your skin will turn yellow. Stones can also go to the pancreas and lead to pancreatitis (inflamation of the pancreas).

B-12 – B-12 cannot be taken through the stomach. It can be attained by injection or taken sublingually to be absorbed. However, it can be attained naturally from eating meat. When B-12 is taken from protein in meat it does so through the "intrinsic factor" on the way to being absorbed by the intestines.

Sulfur – plentiful in onions, garlic, eggs, and nuts. It is a form of B-1, which is good for bones, hair, skin and connective tissue. Sulphur is needed for strong cell membranes (collagen). Vegetarians usually are deficient in sulfur.

Vitamin A – good for cell collagen, eyes, skin and the teeth.

Vitamin B1–helps glucose metabolize and it has neurological benefits that aid memory cells.

Vitamin B3--A detoxifier that helps to produce stomach acid, while it lowers cholesterol levels and dilates the blood vessels.

Vitamin B6 – good for diabetic neuropathy, cell communication and cellular heath. Also, Biotin, part of B-vitamin complex, helps to maintain healthy hair and it also aids in body growth.

Vitamin C–helps to repair and protect cell membranes (collagen).

Vitamin D–helps to detox cell waste and absorb calcium.It also helps to reduce obesity.

Vitamin E –Free radical fighter in fatty tissue.

CHAPTER SIX

(Various ailments and diseases and ways to combat them)

Acne--Acne–should be dealt with internally, because acne originates from an internal dysfunction that triggers the outbreak.

→**Acne can be caused by:** a hormone imbalance, low progesterone; a vitamin and mineral deficiency; insufficient amount of fatty acids; low thyroid; Poor digestion; toxins in the blood and liver stones. Also, if you have low progesterone, along with a deficiency of Vitamin A, the combination may ignite an acne outbreak. In conjunction, if a person has a low thyroid condition and a deficiency in Vitamin A, along with low progesterone, it may cause the body not to convert cholesterol to progesterone, which would cause acne.

Excessive sugar in the diet can start the production of androgens. The excessive sugar arouses the sebaceous gland which then produces skin cells that cause the pores of the skin to accumulate bacteria. The accumulation of bacteria blocks the pores and creates the acne. Another cause of acne is poor nutrition. To help avoid low nutrition, take multivitamins and colloidal trace minerals.

Diets that aid in fighting acne:

→Diets consisting of only raw fruit, raw vegetables, fish, free range meats, and poultry can prevent acne; however, it is imperative that the diet contains no processed foods. Acne is more prevalent in western civilization due to the popular but unhealthy diets such as fast-foods, frozen foods, white flour, over-processed food (referred to as dead foods) and grain fed animals; the latter may contain antibiotics, hormones and other chemicals.

Supplementation is also necessary to provide the body with the necessary resources necessary to resolve the acne problem from the inside of the body.

These supplemental resources include:

After washing your face, apply lemon juice and make a paste composed of bentonite clay and apple cider vinegar. Leave the mask (clay and vinegar) on for at least one hour. The process will help in detoxification. Another old time remedy is the combination of honey and oatmeal mixed into a paste to act as a mask. Place the mask on your face and leave it in place for about one hour before washing it off. Also, a facial wash with the combination of Witch Hazel, the herb yarrow and nettle tincture can be helpful. Another topical application that may be used is Milk of Magnesium.

Other sources: Multivitamin and Colloidal Minerals take as directed by label; colloidal silver, a mineral which is applied topically, contains antibacterial and anti-microbial properties; Herbal tea (Goldenseal aids in fighting bad bacteria); Essential fatty acids of flaxseed; fish oil; Zinc; B complex vitamin; Calcium; magnesium; onions (the sulphur in onions helps the healing process); oregano oil; chromium (helps regulate the blood sugar); milk thistle (helps to detox the liver) and selenium (a trace mineral).

Styptic pencils, used topically, will kill bacteria and help to dry up oily skin. The pencil contains sulphur which absorbs oil. The topical use of natural progesterone cream is also helpful along with taking zinc on a daily basis may also be helpful. Some other sources of help against acne include topical Vitamin A, Witch Hazel, tea tree oil and lavender oil used in combination (mixed in a bottle) can be patted on the areas where the acne is visible and yet another source is Neem oil (apply topically), which is rich in guercetin and is antibacterial and antifungal. Nevertheless, remember that topical treatment cannot work without the detoxification process and a proper diet. It is important to note that in some cases, high dosages of Vitamin A have cured acne; however, high doses should only be taken for a limited period of time, particularly if you are or intend to get pregnant.

Alzheimer's disease –This condition could be caused by a loss of Myelin, which is the layer of insulation that protects the nerve cells in the brain and the spinal cord. Myelin, composed of fatty substances and protein, covers and protects the nerve cells. It also controls the speed of the impulses that travels along the nerve cells. If the myelin becomes damaged, the speed of the nerve impulses decreases and that can lead to other diseases, including multiple sclerosis.

Damage to the myelin is also caused by the aging process and a slowdown in using the brain. However, aging does not automatically cause less activity in the brain. Keeping active, reading, learning new skills including how to use a computer can stimulate the body to create new brain cells. Another cause of the loss of myelin is linked to a deficiency in the immune system such as hypoglycemia, or disorder in the thyroid gland, and even vitamin and mineral deficiencies.

Another cause could be a toxin buildup, such as aluminum, in the system which might affect the health of the brain. Aluminum is contained in some antiperspirants, pharmaceuticals and cooking utensils. Detoxification is a good beginning and it is also helpful to take supplements such as, multivitamins, Colloidal Minerals, fish oil and magnesium.

It is also important to refrain from white flour, white sugar, processed foods and grain-fed red meat. Other foods that should be avoided include dairy products and over-cooked food, which destroys the enzymes that are the foundation of the immune system. It is also important to avoid food enhancers, including msg (which contain excessive glutamate), called excitotoxins. The excitotoxins are due to the excessive glutamate, which causes the brain cells to die through a process known as apoptosis (cell death).

In one hypothesis it is thought that if a person is hypoglycemic (loss of glucose to the brain) it allows glutamate to be excessive in the brain, which causes cell death. Another hypothesis is that people suffering with Alzheimer's disease also suffer from hyper-phosphation (too much phosphate to nerve cells).

→–eliminate processed foods, carbonated drinks and non-free range meats.

→detox liver and blood to get rid of those toxins.

→take lithium, one of many minerals in Colloidal Minerals which will inhibit hyper-phosphation.
→Take the herb turmeric, a multi-vitamin and Vitamin B-12. The B-12 should be taken separately from the multivitamin because it is only absorbable when placed under the tongue (sublingually).

Other suggestions or options that can be tried: MCT medium chain triglycerides, commonly found in coconut oil, are being used to treat Alzheimer's because it is known that the cocoanut oil is an energy source that does not require insulin to gain access to the brain cells.

→Club Moss (Chinese herb)–used with alpha-lipoic acid to enhance memory.
→Ginkgo biloba–an ancient herb that enhances memory because it dilates the blood vessels.

In addition, take a multivitamin supplement and colloidal trace minerals supplements and niacinamide (Vitamin B-3); blueberries eat plenty and the herb gotukola.

Red Grapes and red wine are both antioxidants and they have the ability to help clear arteries. The French people are known for having diets of rich foods and a high consumption of wine. Nonetheless, the French have low cardiovascular problems and the number of French people who suffer from Alzheimer's disease is also low.

→The herb periwinkle which helps to increase blood flow to the brain. Periwinkle, which has been used by Europeans for centuries, also contains alkaloids, which help to protect the brain cells from sustaining damage.
→ The herb turmeric aids in circulation. Exercise helps to improve circulation and drinking sage tea is also beneficial to circulation.
→ Calcification of the arteries, a form of heart disease, which may cause a lower blood supply. It can be the result of a deficiency of Vitamin K-3 and magnesium.

→Eating nuts is very helpful in the struggle with Alzheimer's and of the nut family, walnuts, which are rich in Omega 3, have gained a reputation of being very helpful. They are frequently referred to as the perfect "brain food."

→Another strong item known to aid in the fight against Alzheimer's disease is organic apple juice, known to help prevent oxidation, which triggers the accumulation of plaque. Plaque buildup is common in people who suffer from Alzheimer's disease. The supplement lutein may be helpful in reducing plaque build-up. Also, taking Vitamin E in high doses may help to slow the progression of the disease.

→The enzyme known as Luteolin fights toxins that have entered the brain. It is found in carrots, celery, olive oil, peppers, spices.

→Another product, Zeolite (mineral) is available over the counter at local health stores. It works to detoxify heavy metals. Bentonite clay, mixed with water, aids in cellular health by trapping toxic metals and eliminating them from the body.

Doctor Brian McDonough, a medical reporter for KYW News Radio in Philadelphia in his medical report on 13 April, 2010 stated: "A diet of salad, nuts, poultry, fruits and vegetables as well as fish reduced the risk of Alzheimer's disease." He also reported that "those foods are rich in vitamins B-12, Vitamin E and folate as reported from the archives of Neurology."

→Protect nerve cells–take ginger and the herb gotu-kola, skullcap turmeric and cinnamon. Other herbs include ginkgo biloba and sage.

→Asian ginseng–take to help protect nerves and to help lower blood sugar. It also helps to improve circulation.

ANEMIA (low iron count)--Low iron means low hemoglobin (part of red blood cells) that carry oxygen. About twenty percent of women, are deficient in iron; however, among pregnant women, the percentage rises to about fifty percent. Men, rarely become iron-deficient.

Iron deficiencies can be corrected by eating food rich in "heme iron," the only type of iron that the body can absorb. Foods rich in iron include the following: shrimp, baked potatoes, beans, beef, chicken, oysters, sardines, and chicken liver.

Ironically spinach and other plants which contain iron is a type called non-heme which is not very absorbable by the body. Cooking in cast iron pans also helps iron deficiencies. It is also important for the blood to be alkaline and for you to limit stress. See booklet chapter on PH on pages 8-9. Also, toxic blood that contains heavy metals can also cause low iron. See Chapter Two on detox of heavy metals using bentonite clay.

Angina–Angina (a type of heart disease)–This condition exists when insufficient blood is flowing to the heart and the most likely cause is due to the arteries being restricted, which makes it imperative that circulation of the blood must be improved. Steps required to increase circulation include the elimination of white sugar, processed carbohydrates, white flour products and white rice. They are basically detrimental and they provide no nutrition. It is equally important that you eliminate red meat from your diet because most animals are grain fed and the grain contains high Omega 6 fat, along with being acidic to the blood. Arteries and blood vessels aid in circulation and they are enhanced by a diet that includes garlic, Hawthorne tea, herbal teas, a good multivitamin, Colloidal Minerals, Coenzyme Q10 and magnesium.

→ **Omega 3** (fish oil) D-Ribose (take as prescribed on bottle) which helps stop angina and the supplement creatine helps build heart tissue. Elderly people usually have low levels of zinc. It is suggested that people in that category should take extra zinc in addition to taking a multivitamin.

→ Fresh beets help oxygenize the cells. Hawthorne tea, multi herb tea, lots of green vegetables for vitamin and minerals. The amino acid arginine (take as directed) relaxes the arteries, fish oil, coenzyme Q10, wheat germ and Vitamin C.

→A person suffering from angina requires a diet that consists of fruit, vegetables, legumes and high fiber foods Refrain from eating vegetable oils, margarine, fried foods and fast-foods. Mineral deficiencies are common in people who have angina. They need colloidal trace minerals as part of their daily diet and they also require photonutrients (fruits and vegetables). Also, it is necessary to get protein, which is contained in chicken, fish and yogurt. However, it is important that you avoid processed foods, margarine, salt, sugar and processed meats.

→**Celery** contains enzymes that are effective in helping to clear the arteries. Celery should be eaten on a daily basis. The enzymes also work to relax the arteries and dilate the blood vessels. Garlic also helps to clear the blood vessels. Because of its natural anti-viral and anti-microbial activity, garlic also acts as a blood purifier, while it promotes the formation of new blood vessels. The usefulness of both celery and garlic dates back centuries when they were used as ancient Chinese remedies. Other helpful supplements include:

→**Niacin**, which dilates blood vessels. It can be obtained over the counter and should be taken as directed. The product is called ENDUR.

→**Magnesium**–take as directed.

→**Licthin**–helps to remove artery plaque.

→**Fish oil** –anti-arrhythmic.

→ **Coenzyme Q10**–helps to strengthen the heart. Take as directed on label.

→**L Carnitine**–helps to extract energy from the blood and transport that energy to the cells.

→**L-Arginine**–produces nitric oxide, which dilates the arteries. It is also used as a substitute for Viagra. It should be taken (eight grams per day) on an empty stomach before meals and spread out during the day; rather than taking all at one time.

→**Flaxseed**–1/4 cup of ground flaxseed daily.

→**Hawthorne** herb–helps the heart to function.

→**DHEA**–take as directed.

Anxiety–A good herbal nerve tonic is a combination of herbs, including skullcap, valerian root, lemon balm, aswagandha and the tops of oats. This is a tea that will help to change your mood from melancholy to positive. Also skullcap is a powerful tonic for the nervous system. Three teaspoons of skullcap root mixed with one cup of water and drink as a cup of tea. You can substitute by using the skullcap root in tincture (takes as directed).

Anxiety is much more common in women; however, men are also affected. Anxiety usually follows a traumatic event and can near instantly change a person's personality. One of the major effects is the loss of self-confidence, which is responsible for transforming an otherwise outgoing gregarious person into a recluse. Another effect is claustrophobia and yet another is the exaggerated fear of the unknown.

Some people, who lack an understanding of how anxiety can be overwhelming, suddenly come to believe that they might be losing their sanity; however, anxiety does not cause insanity. Nevertheless, it is a frightening condition. Once a person inflicted by the condition realizes the scope of the challenge to overcome anxiety, it becomes achievable; however, it is a slow process for many. Once the anxiety is identified and the person realizes that the road to victory lies in restoring self confidence, the road to success is at hand.

Symptoms of anxiety include the following: Heart palpitations; Sweaty palms; exaggerated fearfulness; fear of travel; fear of committing suicide; fear of going insane; fear of hearing bad news; fear of being alone; fear of making a decision, even minor decisions and fear of being in crowds.

Anxiety (panic) attacks occur unexpectedly, but rarely during a time when a clear head is required; rather, they emerge well after the crisis occurs. Amazingly, while engaged in the battle of overcoming anxiety, a person who attempts to bring on an attack fails. Proper treatment and patience, along with a proper diet can shorten the length of time required to overcome the anxiety, but it can be beaten, once a person begins to be willing to restore self-confidence. Once an anxiety attack passes and the person begins to realize that the exaggerated fear was baseless, it will become more clear that anxiety can be cured with persistence.

Arrhythmia–Take fish oil on a daily basis and also take Superoxide Dismutase daily. The Superoxide Dismutase will increase the amount of oxygen in the blood and repair cells damaged through oxidation. It is thought by some that arrhythmia is caused by a copper deficiency. Take the supplement copper, along with magnesium.

Arthritis:

→ Arthritis–There are many types of arthritis and it can be caused by various things, including a body's acidic environment.

→Excess body fat can put stress on joints and old injuries.

→Food allergies and a lack of digestive tract bacteria can contribute to arthritis.

The Types of Arthritis include:

→**Osteoarthritis**--caused by the degeneration of the large, weight-bearing joints of the body.

→**Rheumatoid Arthritis**–which is caused by auto-immune conditions, when a person's immune system attacks its own joints. The joints that most often become affected are the smaller joints of the hands. They become tender and swollen, and the arthritis can also cause the hands to become deformed.

→ **Gout--**a form of arthritis caused by a buildup of uric acid in the body. It is produced by the breakdown of substances known as purines, which are found in all of the body's tissues; however, purines are also found in a variety of foods, including anchovies, dried beans, liver, peas and shellfish. Usually, uric acid dissolves in the blood and after passing through the kidneys it exits the body through urine. Nonetheless, the buildup of uric acid in the blood can be caused by the body which naturally produces uric acid, but fails to excrete it through the kidneys. Rather, the uric acid enters the joints and crystalizes. Once the uric acid crystalizes, it causes pain. Another cause of the buildup of uric acid is due to the diet, particularly when a person excessively eats foods that are high in purines. Also, the condition can sometimes be traced to heredity.

High levels of uric acid in the blood is known as hyperuricemia; however, the condition does not automatically result in gout attacks; rather, most people who have high levels of the uric acid do not suffer from gout unless the condition causes uric acid crystals to form in the body.

People more susceptible to suffer from gout include, primarily men who have a family history of gout, however, others include men who are overweight or drink alcoholic beverages excessively. Others include men or women whose diets are rich in purines. In conjunction, enzymes are required to break down purines. If an individual has an enzyme deficiency, the body must struggle to break down the purines. If you are suffering from gout, it is important that you consume large amounts of raw foods, or lightly cooked foods, which contain more enzymes.

The causes of gout attacks vary. Gout attacks can be caused by alcohol or drugs, but an attack can be traced to stress and even from a separate illness. Most attacks last from about three to ten days, with or without treatment. A subsequent gout attack is difficult to predict. It could be months or sometimes years before a person suffers a re-occurrence.

Gout is known to be among the most painful types of arthritis. Once the buildup occurs, the uric acid can lead to:

→ uric acid crystal deposits in joints (frequently occurs in the big toe).

→ Deposits of uric acid (called tophi) that appear to resemble lumps under the skin.

→ Kidney stones caused by uric acid crystals in the kidneys.

In many cases, gout initially occurs in a person's big toe, which becomes "very sore, red, warm, and swollen." Gout can also affect ankles, elbows, fingers, heels, knees and wrists.

→ Recommended foods- flaxseed and cold water fish (salmon and mackerel) have anti-inflammatory properties. Eat lots of raw vegetables and whole grains to sweep away minerals and acid build up as well as to keep your digestive system free of harmful bacteria. Broccoli and cauliflower are especially helpful.

→Need good PH (Alkalinity) as it affects cartilage growth and nutrient absorption. Also, the body needs the antioxidants contained in raw fruits and vegetables to help stop free radicals that can cause various types of arthritis. Good Ph is also achieved by taking a little helping of baking soda, mixed with water on a daily basis. It helps to keep the urinary tract alkaline, while it reduces uric acid levels.

Foods that are high in sulfur such as; asparagus, cabbage, garlic, or onions eaten everyday help to repair cartilage and bone. Also, drink lots of water to help rid the body of toxins and prevent dehydration, which is also associated with arthritis. Also, raw pineapple contains an enzyme called Bromelain, which helps to reduce inflamation.

Avoid foods that are acidic, saturated fats, fried foods, dairy, refined carbohydrates, pasta, bread, caffeine, meat, eggs, refined sugars and man made sweeteners.

Some foods such as tomatoes, potatoes, eggplant, and peppers, all of which contain the ingredient, solanine can trigger allergic or arthritic-like reactions. Eliminate these night-shade vegetables for about six weeks to see if there is any improvement.

Supplements to take include Glucosamine sulfate (helps to reduce joint pain and rebuild cartilage). It can also be taken with Condroitin; MSM, an anti-inflammatory that contains sulfur, an integral part of cartilage; fish oil contains three fatty acids that reduce joint inflammation and helps promote joint lubrication. High potency multivitamins, rich in antioxidants, help to prevent joint tissue destruction. Take as directed on container. Jell-O or gelatin contains the same ingredients as chicken bone marrow and is considered a great source of cartilage-like properties that help to protect the joints.

Gout (Remedies)

One old remedy for gout is a combination of raw honey and apple cider vinegar taken between meals. The combination will help to remove uric acid that enters the joints. An accumulation of uric acid in the body, due to either heredity or from a bad diet, can create problems because the kidneys are unable to dispose of the excess acid. Also, a small amount of baking soda, mixed with water, taken in the morning before breakfast helps to eliminate uric acid and it helps to keep the bladder alkaline.

Other old time remedies that are helpful against gout include orange juice, which contains potassium; pineapple, which contains bromelain (can also be found in capsule form) and the supplement Quercetin; the foods and the supplement Quercetin each work to suppress the accumulation of uric acid. Other supplements that are useful include Vitamin E, flaxseed oil and black cherry concentrate.

Uric acid is a necessary antioxidant in the body, however, if levels rise, the acid crystallizes and results in joint pain and kidney problems. Usually, the condition is a precursor to diabetes. A simple remedy that can be helpful is to eat large amounts of bing cherries or drink substantial portions of blackberry juice. Nonetheless, caution is required because of the high amount of sugar fructose which is contained in fruit. It is also helpful to drink olive leaf teas (often) or use the supplement olive leaf extract. Olive leaf teas and also the extract both work to lower blood pressure and blood sugar.

Olive leaf was used for medicinal purposes as far back as Biblical times and was actually noted in "Ezekiel 47:12." Celery stalks and celery seed extract are also helpful. Take the extract as directed on label or eat three stalks of celery every day. The process in lowering blood pressure is not instant; rather, it takes about six month before you see the results. Celery is also instrumental in reducing uric acid because it is a diuretic; however, celery does not alter the balance of potassium and sodium. Simultaneously, the celery or celery seed extract inhibits the build-up of uric acid. For More Information on Gout and other related conditions, see the following website: http://www.niams.nih.gov/Health_Info/Gout/gout_ff.asp.

Arthritis can be recognized in many forms, including joint pain, back pain and bad knees. However, often these problems, although thought of as being arthritis, are not arthritis. Sometimes, the cause of the problem is related to dehydration a condition that has become rampant in our fast-moving society. One sure method to prevent dehydration and rule it out as a symptom of arthritis is to drink lots of water every day. By drinking plenty of water you also help to detoxify your body and you ensure that you have the synovial fluid in your joints, which originates from the water you drink.

Another form of pain that resembles arthritis pain is that which is caused by the calcification of the joints due to excessive calcium in the diet and insufficient magnesium, the latter being necessary to keep the calcium in the blood liquid. It is important to add magnesium to the diet and or cut back on calcium supplements. Over calcium supplementation is common and it can cause the calcium to appear in arteries and in the heart.

To relieve arthritis symptoms, drink Bragg's apple cider vinegar mixed with water and honey. Add two teaspoons of vinegar and two teaspoons of unprocessed honey to a glass of water, and drink this three times a day. The combination helps to keep PH high and it reduces the pain of arthritis. You can also replace the liquid vinegar with natural apple cider vinegar tablets, but be sure to also drink a large amount of water daily.

Once the pains that resemble arthritis have been identified and eliminated, it becomes imperative to begin to focus on the ways to prevent, reduce and even eliminate authentic arthritis. As previously mentioned, arthritis can be triggered by various causes, including acidosis (acidic blood); digestive problems (lack of enzymes and or good bacteria); allergic reactions to specific foods. Another major factor is being overweight. Common unhealthy diets and excessive body fat becomes the precursor to various ailments including arthritis. Yet another cause of arthritis originates due to a deficiency in sulphur levels or acidic blood (low PH).

People who suffer from Arthritis usually have acidic blood, which makes it important that they eat more alkaline foods (fruits and vegetables); however refrain from eating barley, eggplant, peppers, tomatoes, parsley and meat. It is equally important that you keep your stress level low. High stress causes an interruption of the proteins that feed the cells, which in turn, may cause cell mutation.

Once the arthritis is identified, it becomes imperative that you begin to change your unhealthy diet to a well-balanced healthy diet. After beginning your new diet, the next step is to try the following remedies:

Joint Pain-If you experience joint pain, it may help if you lower sugar intake (blood sugar) and simultaneously add cod liver oil, which contains Omega3, to your diet.

Arthritis Fighters

➔**Anti-inflammatory Herbs**

➔**Bioflavonoids**–It is recommended that you eat (daily) the following to reduce inflamation: dark fruit that contains pits, green tea, onions, berries and whole grains, Omega fatty acids- reduce inflammation.

➔**Boron**-Helps to keep the calcium in your bones. Boron is also found in beans, green leaf vegetables, grapes and nuts.

➔**Boswella (**herb)--Boswella is anti-inflammatory. Take as directed.
➔ **Bromelain**-a good anti-inflammatory, is also found in pineapples.
➔**Devil's claw**–Helps to reduce arthritis pain, as reported by a British researcher and published in Phytotherapy Research. Take as directed on a daily basis.
➔**Fish Oil** -Good for joints. It is also an anti-inflammatory. Herring, mackerel, salmon and sardines contain high amounts of fish oil.
➔**Flaxseed Oil**--Lessens inflammation.
➔**Hyaluric Acid**–A joint lubricant that aids in cartilage. Take as directed.
➔**Magnesium**–helps to keep calcium liquid, which stops calcium from hardening the arteries and joints of the body.
➔**Niacinamide**--dilates blood vessels and increases circulation.
➔**Selenium**--Selenium is found in garlic, meats, oatmeal, oysters, shrimp, swordfish, tuna, cracked wheat bread and sunflower seeds.
➔**Tripterygium Wilfordii Hook f**– an extract herb.
➔**Turmeric**–an antioxidant–use large amounts of the herb turmeric on your food.
➔**Vitamin A--**Carotenoids (take as directed) are found in yellow and orange fruits and vegetables such as apricots, cantaloupe, carrots, mangoes and sweet potatoes and also in dark leafy vegetables including broccoli, collard greens, parsley and spinach.
➔**Vitamin C**–found in: broccoli, brussel sprouts, cabbage, cantaloupe, grapefruit, mangoes, oranges, potatoes, raspberries and red peppers. Vitamin C is also available as a supplement.
➔**Vitamin E**–found in asparagus, whole grain breads, broccoli, cereals, nuts, peaches, peanut butter, spinach, sunflower seeds, vegetable oils and wheat. Vitamin E is also available as a supplement.
➔**Exercise**–Exercise is important because it increases circulation, while it aids in detoxification.
➔**Low sulphur levels or low PH**--Eggs, garlic and onions. Also, may be caused due to a need for the minerals copper and or zinc.

Wearing a copper bracelet is also helpful. Vitamin B-3, which opens blood vessels is also helpful. Sulphur compounds rebuild cartilage and they also aid in eliminating toxins. Sulphur compounds also help to detoxify the liver by helping to produce glutathione.

➔**Cod liver oil**–An old time supplement for Vitamin D and Omega 3. Cod liver oil is considered by some to be more helpful for joints than fish oil; take as directed. Cod liver oil is also good for Rheumatoid arthritis, however, the dosage is higher (8,000 mg daily–Prevention Magazine September 2008, page 54). Cod Liver Oil is often referred to as Grandma's cure. It is best to take cod liver oil on an empty stomach.

➔**Herbs** increase blood supply to joints to keep down inflammation.

➔**Celery**–Eat plenty of celery every day to increase circulation, and to open up the blood vessels. Celery is also good for reducing cholesterol. A supplement for celery, celery seed is available over the counter.

➔**Omega 3 and flax seed oil**–You can also achieve the same results by eating more fish. Eskimos do not normally get Arthritis due to their cold water fish diet, which is full of Omega 3. Omega 3 (contained in fish oil) helps to lubricate the body's joints.

➔**Vitamin E** - prevent tissue damage of Arthritis.

➔**Jell-O** - eat daily, this has same properties as cartilage.

➔**Meat broth** –good for joints.

➔**Pumpkin seed oil** - reduces inflammation and it is also good for prostate swelling.

➔**Coral calcium**--The best source of calcium. It prevents osteoporosis. Take in combination with magnesium.

➔**Black Cherry juice** - reduces inflammation. Drink before eating things that will bring on Gout or Gout symptoms such as swelling.

➔**Alfalfa tablets**–The alfalfa tablets contain high amounts of nutrients.

➔**Fruits and vegetables** –both help to clean out acid and detox the body. Fruits and vegetables also contain needed nutrients and antioxidants.

➔**Vegetables and foods to avoid**-- Night shade vegetable (asparagus, beans, cauliflower, egg plant, peppers, potatoes and tomatoes. You should also avoid bacon and organ meats. In conjunction, the caution on food to avoid is pointed toward those who are allergic to the poisons that are naturally produced to shield themselves from the insects that attack them.

➔**Water consumption** –drink lots of water daily to flush toxins out of your kidneys and liver. Water is also important to keep your joints hydrated.

➔**Ginger**–eat ginger, either the raw herb or tincture in water.

➔**Green Tea**–This tea is anti-inflammatory which reduces the production of prostaglandins (pain messengers).

➔**Herbal tea (multi)** –Helps circulation in the entire body and aids in detoxification.

→**Hibiscus Flower Tea** –Loaded with Vitamin C. It also raises HDL.

→**Pineapple** –contains Bromelain a natural pain killer.

→**Herbs**–Sage, turmeric, ginger, cayenne and Gotu Kola. All are anti-inflammatory.

→**Hot peppers**–hot peppers contain capsican and cayenne pepper, both of which block pain signals.

Supplements that may be taken:

→(**Option 1**) Sea lipped mussels and gelatin capsules. Take as directed.

→(**Option 2**) Drunken raisins–A legendary treatment. Place yellow raisins in a pint of Gin. After four days, strain the excess liquid and place the raisins in a glass jar. Eat nine of the raisins with your morning meal. There is no evidence that the "drunken raisins" will cure arthritis; however, they contain anti-inflammatory ingredients.

→**(Option 3**) Cat's claw herb.

→(**Option 4**) Make some tea from cucumber magnolia bark (two cups), prickly ash bark (one cup), Black cohosh (one cup), Wild yam (one cup) and Wild cherry bark (one cup).

→ (**Option 5**)–Omega 3 and flaxseed are anti-inflammatory. Eat raw vegetables and fruit to fight acid buildup and unwanted bacteria. Vegetables including asparagus, cabbage, garlic and onions contain sulphur, an anti-inflammatory agent. Pineapples also contain an anti-inflammatory ingredient, bromelain. Avoid acidic foods such as; fried foods, dairy products, white bread, white flour, meat and eggs. Also nightshade vegetables such as eggplant, tomatoes and peppers can cause arthritis to flare up. Supplements should include: boron, chondroitin; fish oil; gelatin; glucosamine sulphate and a multivitamin, to help prevent arthritis. Selenium. Flaxseed oil, Vitamin A, Vitamin C and Vitamin E are also helpful supplements.

→(**Option 6**)–Eat more eggs, which are known as the "world's most perfect food."

→ **(Option 7)**–The supplement red seaweed reduces pain caused by inflammation. Calcium and magnesium helps to curb inflamation and increase bone density.

Rheumatoid Arthritis--An autoimmune system failure takes place when your body's own immune system attacks the body's joint tissue. Is can also be the result of allergies, infection or bad bacteria in the intestinal tract. A body full of toxins, especially heavy metals, such as mercury, can be a contributing factor. In addition, an acidic body can also cause problems with the immune system.

Dietary supplements should be taken to treat Rheumatoid Arthritis, similarly to general arthritis. However, to help eliminate some of the above issues, try the following:

→ Detoxification: See Chapter Two.

→ Remove bad bacteria from the intestines by using Oregano oil (P73), raw garlic, a probiotic (yogurt or sauerkraut).

→ Keep an alkaline body. Use apple cider vinegar and refer to Chapter One regarding PH.

Try to narrow down food that might trigger an allergic reaction and check for possible airborne causes. Follow the dietary supplements in the arthritis section. This includes fish oil, vitamins, Colloidal Minerals, condroitin and gluclosamine with MSM gelatin tablets and lipid sea muscles, to name a few. Some others are: Cod liver oil, zinc, copper, selineum, B-12 and Vitamin C. Also, eliminate nightshade vegetables, which can trigger Rheumatoid Arthritis symptoms.

Eliminate soda or other phosphoric foods, as it leaches calcium from the bones and sends it into the blood. This may cause the calcium to collect in the joints and trigger the parathyroid gland which will add more calcium to the blood.

Several herbs that may also help, are: yucca roots, pepper, turmeric, horsetail (for its silica), ginger, devils claw and boswella. Also, an ancient Chinese herb (Triptolide, also known as Thunder god vine) can help by reducing the bad cells in the DNA.

Age Spots–may be caused by a poor antioxidant diet or a vitamin and colloidal mineral deficiency, however, the condition can also be caused by bad fats in the diet or excess overcooked foods. The overcooked foods causes the destruction of the enzymes the body requires to function properly. Another item, charred barbeque food, is considered to be dead food and the carbon created by charring the food creates HCA's, which may be carcinogenic. Also detox (See Chapter Two) is necessary to keep the body free of toxins and to protect the liver. Castor oil applied to spots may also help.

→(**Detox**)–herbal tea with one drop of lavender or bentonite clay in water. The herb milk thistle is also useful in detoxification. It also adds a protective coating on the liver. Also, take selenium and Vitamin E.

Aging--The supplements Carnitine and lipoic acid enhance the cellular use of fatty acids. They also work to decrease cell damage that otherwise leads to aging. Also, Lipoic acid is helpful in breaking down fatty acids, while it works to increase cellular energy by increasing glutathione, an antioxidant that helps to remove cell waste from the body.

Ankles, Swollen–A swollen ankle is a sign of poor circulation. The herb Job's tears and parsley are diuretics that help to reduce swelling in the ankles.

Arteriosclerosis –The arteries become affected by Arteriosclerosis and it is caused by plaques that accumulate in the medium and large arteries. The plaques including fats and cholesterol, collect along the walls of the affected coronary arteries to impede the free flow of blood to the heart. Bragg's apple vinegar and raw honey also helps.

This condition, once the arteries become more narrow, can slow or even block the steady flow. Shortness of breath or chest pain (angina) may develop or other symptoms including leg pains and swelling of the legs. If you suffer from this disorder, you will notice that the more you move around, the leg pain will intensify due to poor circulation.

To do a quick check, press your skin with one of your fingers. If the spot you pressed remains indented, it is a sign that you have arteriosclerosis. Also, some supplements that may be taken include: celery, garlic, lecithin, Colloidal Minerals, fruits and vegetables. A high fiber diet is the key to help clear Arteriosclerosis and helps to eliminate excess cholesterol.

Asthma–Asthma, a word derived from a Greek verb, "aazein," meaning pant, is a chronic lung disease that affects children and adults, primarily in the western countries. Millions of Americans suffer from asthma. A study (Morbidity and Mortality Weekly Report) reported that during 1996, about "10.2 million adults living in the United States have asthma. During June 2010, the U.S.

government (NIH Osteoporosis and Related Bone Diseases National Resources) stated that the number of people presently suffering from Asthma has skyrocketed to more than 22 million and of those, about six million are children.

People who suffer from asthma can suffer an attack at any time and the attacks can be triggered by many different things, including animals, certain foods, chemicals, emotional distress, dust, food preservatives, infections, perfume and even exercise. Everyone reacts differently and attacks vary from mild to severe.

The symptoms of asthma include: Difficulty in breathing; Coughing (In the case of children, a dry cough might develop or their chest begins to itch); Rapid Heart Beat; Excessive sweating; Tightening of the chest and Wheezing.

Trying to detect the exact causes of asthma is often difficult; however, it is necessary to try to pinpoint what brings on the attack. An attack triggered by food is the rarest of the causes. Nevertheless, if a food is the cause, it is more likely that is the food preservative used in the product.

Many people who suffer from asthma are convinced that their bouts with asthma originate with their diets, particularly dairy products. Nonetheless, sometimes, a person who believes that milk and other dairy products trigger their attacks discover that the cause was tied to an allergic reaction to the dairy products. One other major concern centers around children who suffer from asthma. Often children with asthma do not eat dairy products or drink milk due to some apprehension about triggering an attack, but in that case, the children are being deprived from receiving the necessary calcium that their bones require to aid the growing process by building strong bones.

It is extremely helpful if a person who begins to suffer from asthma maintains a journal, which will keep a list of when the attacks occur as well as the possible caused. You might want to consider your day's activities as well as the foods you ate on that particular day. The journal should also include the environmental conditions that existed.

The following is a list of some foods and preservatives that are typically known for triggering an asthma attack:

Foods: Chocolate; Citrus Fruits; Coffee; Corn; Dairy products; Eggs; Fish, including shellfish; Milk; Peanuts; Peppermint; Tomatoes and Wheat.

Preservatives and other things that might cause an asthma attack:

→FD&C Yellow 5 (tartrazine), a food coloring; however, it is also used in other products including shampoo and various personal care products and in many condiments, such as salt and mustard.

→Monosodium glutamate--a flavor enhancer found in fast-foods along with frozen dinners. Other products in which it is found can include packaged soups and sauces including soy sauce, steak sauce and Worcestershire sauce. Yet other causes that could trigger an asthma attack include Bird Feathers; Chemical vapors; Dehydration; Dust Mites; Genetics; Pollen and stress. Poor digestion can also cause an attack if undigested food enters the intestinal tract, which could cause poor nutrient assimilation and constipation. Dander from animals, particularly cats is also known to be a source of attacks. When a cat licks its hair, it leaves a protein on the hair and from there the protein becomes airborne and easily is absorbed into a person's blood.

There is no known cure for asthma. Nonetheless, the condition can be treated and there are various ways that contribute to minimizing attacks, including: drinking substantial amounts of water to prevent dehydration. Water helps to prevent mucus from forming in your body. The diet should consist of raw vegetables, fruits, including apples, which help to keep the airways clear and open. The diet should also be confined to chicken, fish and lean meat, along with garlic and onions, both of which are anti-inflammatory and they contain sulphur. Dairy products should be avoided.

Other items useful in managing asthma, include: B Complex vitamins; Borage oil, which fights inflammation associated with asthma. Take as directed on label; Copper–Relaxes the muscles of the lungs; Fish oil–source of Omega 3; Flaxseed oil; Gingko Biloba (herb)–dilates the blood vessels; Magnesium–Helps relax bronchial tubes; sweet gum; tea of wild plum; trace or Colloidal Minerals–supplies minerals that you are not receiving from food; Turmeric (herb)–antioxidant that helps protect the lungs. Other supplements that help include: Vitamin A, Vitamin C and Vitamin D; wild cherry bark; zinc (mineral); red grapefruit and egg yolks, which contain Vitamin A. All of the above mentioned supplements work to help increase the capacity of the lungs.

Steroid inhalers are used frequently by many people who suffer from asthma attacks; however there is risk involved with long-term use of the inhalers. The risks include side effects such as the loss of bone density and cataracts. One option, rather than a steroid inhaler, would be to use a nasal spray such as Sinu Orega, which is available at local health stores or online. The spray can be combined with oregano oil (P73); use it sublingually (place under the tongue for five minutes, before swallowing).

ADHD (Attention Deficient Disorder)–avoid food coloring–nitrates and sugar-additives because they may interfere with nervous signals. Helpful supplements include Vitamins A, C, D and E, magnesium, folic acid, iodine, fatty acids and a thyroid glandular thytrophin.

Alcohol (Drinking heavily)–Heavy drinking of alcohol lowers glutathione levels in the liver which impedes the liver's part in the detoxification process. Low glutathione levels may also lead to cirrhosis or other liver diseases. Supplement with glutathione and eat foods rich in glutathione such as: brussels sprouts, cauliflower, kale, cabbage, broccoli, asparagus, spinach. The herb turmeric plus omega 3, niacin, (Vitamin B3) help to block triglycerides from forming in the liver. Glutathione also protects against triglycerides forming in the liver.

Anemia–caused by an insufficient amount of iron in the body. The usual cause of a lack of iron is due to a loss of blood or a poorly balanced diet; however, another cause of iron-deficiency anemia occurs due to the body's inability to absorb sufficient amounts of iron from the food.

Low levels of iron in a woman's body can occur due to the loss of blood during the menstrual period or during childbirth. Other causes of blood loss in women is caused by bleeding fibroids in the uterus and bleeding in the urinary tract.

The best sources of iron are meat, poultry, fish, eggs, and iron-fortified foods, the latter having had iron added. If the proper foods are not eaten, the chances of getting iron-deficiency anemia are greatly increased; however, in the United States, iron deficiencies are rare. Foods that are naturally rich in absorbable iron (ferritin) include lima beans, navy beans, red meat and soybeans. If you are going to take an iron supplement, it should be Heme iron.

Also, hefty portions of raw vegetables, especially dark leafy ones, and sauerkraut should be added to the diet. Sauerkraut aids in digestion by adding enzymes in the stomach. The raw vegetables also aid in absorption. One caution, you should not drink carbonated soda because the phosphorous contained in soda depletes the immune system and extracts calcium from the bones. Iron-deficiency anemia is also associated with fatigue and low red or white blood cell count. Blood has a lower amount of oxygen due to fewer red cells.

A poor red cell count signals that the liver is functioning poorly and requires detoxification (See Chapter Two). If the condition exists, the herbs lavender and milk thistle can help. Milk thistle also forms a protective coating on the liver. If you have a low white cell count, it is an indication of a poor immune system. It is necessary to eat more protein, such as meat.

Also, supplements that should be taken include: Colloidal Minerals, which contain copper, selenium and zinc, all of which are necessary to combat a low white cell count. High Potency Multivitamins are also helpful.

Athlete's Foot– Calendula tea, which can be taken internally or it can be applied topically. Calendula tea is anti-bacterial and anti-viral. Other similar treatments include P73 oregano oil or Tee Tree oil. Another helpful treatment is to soak your feet in salt water, including the ocean if you happen to be at a seashore resort. The salt creates a osmotic environment that kills bacteria.

Allergies–An allergy is a reaction of the immune system to something that could be food related or from such things as cosmetics or chemicals. Another cause could be the environment.

The best initial approach is to begin a 5-day fast, which should consist only of fruit juices. If at the end of the 5-day fast, the allergic reaction ceases, you have pinpointed the cause to a food allergy. Some foods designated as causes of allergies include eggs, nuts and shellfish. Nevertheless, if the allergy continues, the cause might be caused by a vitamin or mineral deficiency or a combination of both.

In an effort to eliminate the allergic reaction if it is caused by any of the above reasons, it is recommended that you take a multivitamin and Colloidal Minerals, which can be purchased at a health store. Take as directed on label. Also, other supplements that may be helpful include: Nettle Tincture (helps fight inflamation) and Horehound Tincture (dilates blood vessels). Good stomach bacteria (yogurt, sauerkraut and acidolphilis) helps fight allergies.

Back Problems:

Disc Pain–Could be caused by too many toxins in the body. See Chapter Two on Detoxification. The supplements, Vitamin C, B Complex and calcium may help.

Belly fat to reduce food intake so the body can start to feed off of excess fat take psyllium husks with plenty of water its bulk will keep your appetite down.

Blood Pressure High–A high fiber diet is the key to controlling high blood pressure, because the fiber helps to eliminate cholesterol. Following the suggestions listed below does not instantly bring about positive results; rather, it takes about six months.

→Eat raw vegetables and whole grains (oats, beans, nuts, seed).

→Keep hydrated and drink plenty of water.

→Lower salt intake and increase potassium eat apples asparagus, cabbage, tomatoes, bananas, kelp, alfalfa, onions, raw garlic, parsley and 4 sticks of celery daily. Also, onions and raw garlic are my favorite way to dilate blood vessels and remove artery plaque due to their enzymes and sulfur contents.

→Salt (sodium) causes water retention which puts increase pressure on artery walls.

→Eliminate all processed foods, fast-foods and cheeses.

→Eliminate bad fats (hydrogenated fats, including margarine and refined oil).

→Eliminate sugar and flour.

→Eat organic dandelion greens or parsley(natural diuretics) you can also buy dandelion capsules, which are available over the counter. Take as directed.

→Hawthorne (herb) dilates arteries and reduces high blood pressure. Take as directed.

→Calcium, magnesium and Vitamin D in combination is available. Take as directed.

→Coenzyme Q10 reduces high blood pressure. Take as directed.

→Raw garlic or in capsules form made by Kyolic #106 Garlic Extract. Take as directed.

→Fish oil--Take as directed.

→Potassium--Take as directed. Unpasteurized Apple Cider Vinegar is high in potassium.
→Vitamin C--Take as directed.
→Eliminate sugar, especially white sugar, sometimes referred to as white death.
→Detoxify your body with 1-3 day juice only fast. Make sure the juice contains no sugar. Eating plenty of radishes on a daily basis also helps to detoxify the body.
→Normal blood pressure is below 140/90.
→Colloidal Minerals also known as trace minerals are a must to take.
→A good multi herbal tea relaxes the arteries and provides immune support.
→Vitamin E--incases nitric oxide, which relaxes muscles around the arteries to lower blood pressure and the risk of getting blood clots.
→The herb yarrow dilates blood vessels and lowers blood pressure. The herb yucca powder binds to bad fats and toxins for excretion.
→A western diet condition (high blood pressure)that is much more prevalent in the West than in other parts of the world is due to the types of food that are consumed including: fast foods, overcooked foods, processed foods, grain fed, antibiotic fed and hormone fed fish, meat and poultry. Combine this type of diet with stress, lack of sleep and environmental toxins and you most probably have high blood pressure.
→Resolving HBP is a many fold process. Step 1:detoxification- of toxins, metals and build up of fecal waste. Step 2: a proper diet should include a lot of fiber to get rid of excess cholesterol and keep the digestive tract moving. The foods should include apples with skin, raw vegetables, fruits, beans, nuts, whole grains and yams. When consuming high fiber foods, it is important to remember to drink plenty of water to reduce the chance of becoming constipated.
Add lots of olive oil to the diet, to keep the digestive tract moving. Reduce your intake of salt. While reducing salt, you must increase potassium intake if you consume large amounts of liquid.

Supplements: Vitamin K-2 and magnesium help to stop artery calcification, heel spurs and kidney stones.
Calcium–low levels of calcium can lead to high blood pressure, making it important that you take calcium supplements.
Winter huckleberry tea and Hibiscus flower tea are good for arteries strength and raise HDL.
Grape seed extract (OPC).
Hawthorne herb–contains flavonoids which help to strengthen the blood vessels.
Coenzyme Q10 aids the heart.
L-Carnitine produces nitric oxide to dilate blood vessels.
Vitamin C antioxidant.
Other options:

Blood pressure medicine is all about reducing the amount of the enzyme ACE (Angiotensin) in your blood, which if high, keeps the artery from relaxing and forces the kidney to retain more water and sodium and excrete potassium, which causes the sodium/potassium to become out of balance. The end result is water retention.

Grape seed extract, blueberries and Vitamin K2 act to keep the arteries healthy and elastic, while they also inhibit the enzyme ACE and prevent artery calcification.

Coleus flower herb (dilates blood vessels); dandelion (helps to lower blood pressure); the herb yarrow powder or tincture; Vitamin C; Omega 3 (fish oil) and flax seed are also helpful. Foods that you should include: raw garlic, celery stalks (contain natural enzymes that clear out plaque). In addition, eat foods that are rich in potassium, magnesium and fiber. It is also important that you exercise regularly. It keeps the blood flowing and it dilates the arteries.

Bowels (Irritable Bowl Syndrome-malfunction of digestive tract)–IBS can be caused by stress, fast foods, infection of the digestive tract and poor digestive organs (caused by the lack of good bacteria). It is recommended that you institute a high fiber diet which can include raw carrots, raw vegetables, and lots of water daily;

yogurt and sauerkraut. In conjunction, you receive digestive enzymes from yogurt and sauerkraut. However, you should avoid dairy products, which may trigger IBS. It is equally important that you avoid refined sugar (white) or sweeteners with fructose, flour, red meat, chocolate, caffeine, and spicy foods.

Supplements to take if you are suffering from IBS–Milk thistle; slippery elm (soothes the bowls). Also taking a portion of vinegar (either by drinking or mixing in a salad) before each meal will aid in digestion; digestive enzymes (before each meal); lactobacillus acidophilus (comes in liquid form and helps to prevent harmful microbes from forming in the intestinal tract; enteric-coated peppermint oil capsules (take as directed). Make sure the capsules are enteric-coated. The peppermint oil also helps to reduce cramps and gas. Zinc, an essential mineral, is also helpful for intestinal health.

Also, Chamomile, a multi-purpose herb is also helpful. It calms the intestines, while it fights constipation and diarrhea. Chamomile is available in various forms. Take it in either capsule or tincture as directed after each meal. Another helpful supplement is psyllium seed, which is also a good source of fiber.

Bright's disease–(kidney)-The inflamation of the kidneys could be caused by eating too much protein or from high blood pressure. However, other causes include excessive fluid retention. Blood in the urine is also an indicator of problems with the kidneys. In conjunction, foamy urine which contains blood is a common sign that indicates that a person needs to improve the diet and that herbs should also be taken to supplement the diet. The addition of herbs is extremely helpful in cleansing the bowels and by helping to keep them clean. It is also possible that the condition is caused by heredity.

Herbs and other foods that can be included to improve the diet (with regard to Bright's disease)include:dandelion root (detoxifier); garlic; marshmallow tea (cleanses the kidneys); multi-herbal tea (nutrients); parsley (diuretic); hydrangea (diuretic and kidney cleanser); L-methionine (improves kidney function); L-arginine (dilates blood vessels) and red sumach berries.

Other foods: asparagus; bananas (potassium); digestive enzymes for better digestion; celery; raw cranberries (destroys bad bacteria); lecithin (drink large amounts of water to avoid constipation) watermelon (diuretic).

It is important to refrain from eating sugar, meats, phosphates (soda), dairy products, eggs, and chocolate.

Vitamins and minerals that should supplement the diet include Ionic minerals (trace minerals) and a high potency multi vitamin that contains a high amount of Vitamins A, B, C. E and K, along with zinc and magnesium.

Breast health--iodine is a key element for breast health. Benjamin Eskin MD, an iodine researcher, claims that an iodine deficiency in breast tissue can lead to cancer.

Breath- magnolia bark, as a gum, is an old Chinese remedy that is effective in killing bad bacteria in the mouth. A commercial product, "Eclipse," derived from magnolia bark is also effective in killing bad bacteria.

Bone density–Take DHEA, boron, strontium, calcium, copper, and magnesium to strengthen the bones.

Body pains--Pain (Inflammation) can be the result of an acidic body due to a poor diet. Diets high in carbohydrates, sugar, red meat, and processed foods are acidic and inflammatory. Some people use ibuprofen to relieve pain but fish oil and bromelain (pineapple) do the same thing. Also helpful are raw vegetables, the herbs turmeric, curcumin and herbal tea, green tea. The herb Boswellia can be an effective as an aid plus St. Johns wort, cat's-claw, whit willow bark, arnica, licorice and niacin (vitamin B-3).

Bipolar–Empower Plus, an over the counter product, used to calm pigs is also effective in humans who suffer from a bipolar disorder. Contact a health food store or go online to obtain the product. The mineral lithium (in high doses) may be helpful. It is important that you also take flaxseed oil and Vitamin E to offset the side effects from taking high doses of lithium.

Bloating–Getting a lymph massage is helpful; however, walking, running or general exercise activate the lymph which filters the blood to eliminate toxins (detoxification). Other items that are helpful include: B complex vitamins, bananas and vegetables which contain potassium. You can also add burdock herbal tea as your drink. It is also helpful to cut back on your use of salt.

Bloating usually means poor digestion which requires the initiation of a diet that contains whole foods and a good probotic like acidophilus bifus (digestive enzyme). A good multi herbal tea can also aid in digestion. Ginkgo biloba, gotu kola, Hawthorne and chamomile are good examples of herbal tea. Eating raw sauerkraut or yogurt before meals can also provide the stomach and intestines with good bacteria. Vinegar, taken with water before meals, is beneficial to digestion and it also helps to prevent heartburn. In conjunction, stress causes the reduction of stomach acid. The loss of acid in the stomach causes carbohydrates such as, bread, fruit and juice to ferment, which causes gas.

Blood Pressure (High)–Good pressure is 120/80. When your blood pressure ranges from 120/89 to 139/ 89, it remains acceptable. If your pressure ranges from 140/90 to 145/99; it is borderline high. If your pressure reaches 160/100, you have high blood pressure. Pulse pressure is also important and can be more telling then blood pressure, since it takes into consideration both; 120-80=40, the higher the number the more chance of a heart attack.

Bone health-Astragalus tea helps create macrophoges, which are natural killer cells that attack free radicals by initiating the creation of immune cells in the bone marrow and lymph tissue, where the free radicals cause damage.

Bone spurs- are caused by a calcium deficiency. In addition to taking more calcium, it is also necessary to take Colloidal Minerals, which contain boron, copper and strontium (included in the 74 mineral complex) that works to absorb the calcium. Calcium and magnesium will work to dissolve the spurs, but will take time. It is also important that you use the supplement Vitamin D, which also is needed for calcium to be absorbed.

Bladder problem--Take the herb, three leaf caper, which soothes the bladder lining and supports the sphincters in the bladder. Another option to help keep the bladder healthy and alkaline: mix a small amount of baking soda with water and drink once daily, preferably in the morning. Also, if you are suffering from a bladder cyst, taking baking soda and Bragg's Apple Cider is helpful.

Blood clots– may be caused by a deficiency of Omega 3 (fish oil).

Body odor--armpits are one of the main sources of body odor. It is very helpful to apply tea tree oil before applying a deodorant; however, it might be more helpful if you try a stronger soap before resorting to deodorant. The underarms collect bacteria which becomes the source of the odor. Trying a stronger sop and washing the underarms until you feel certain all the bacteria has been eliminated may be easier on the skin. Deodorants which contain hydrogen peroxide and zinc are known to work well in eliminating underarm body odor. Body odor can also be a sign that you need to detoxify (your body).

Brain health–The loss of brain cells, a natural occurrence during aging causes a reduction in the communication between the cells. The following supplements are helpful: acetyl-L-carnitine and L-dopa, both of which increase metabolism in the brain. Also, Vitamin D and Vitamin B12 both help to guard against brain shrinkage. Vitamin B3 is also helpful because it lowers proteins that are linked to Alzheimer's disease. In addition, folic acid and B6, both function to keep homocysteine levels stable. Fish oil provides the body with fatty acids. The fatty acids are helpful to the brain, which is composed of a large percentage of fat. Cell destruction (oxidation) is always a concern during aging. Vitamin C, Vitamin E and turmeric are antioxidants which combat oxidation. Yet other supplements that may be helpful are ginkgo biloba and the herb vinpocetine. Both help to improve the flow of blood in the brain.

Bursitis pain– Bursitis is related to arthritis. It is the inflamation of the bursas (synovial fluid sacks). The fluid, acting as a lubricant, enables the joints to slide back and forth. However, when the bursas become inflamed, the joints become stiff and pain follows. There is no known cure for bursitis. Taking Vitamin B-12 (as directed on label) is helpful. Other supplements include: cod liver oil (contains Omega 3 and Vitamin D); dark fruit (contain bioflavonoids); fish oil; zinc; gelatin capsules; magnesium, multivitamin; sea mussel capsules; selenium; tumeric and Vitamin C.

Bladder infection–Bladder infections are usually caused in women by E-coli. Cranberry juice and the herb Uva Ursi are both helpful in eliminating bad bacteria. Goldenrod is also helpful along with oregon-grape. They kill bad bacteria including E-coli, while they simultaneously work to prevent bacteria from clinging to bladder walls. Yet another helpful herb is dandelion root extract which helps to eliminate bad bacteria.

Bladder control problems-People suffering from bladder control difficulties may get relief by eating mushrooms, particularly crataeva, ganoderma and shitake. Other options:

Option 1: Chamomile; Chickweed; Cornsilk; Cramp bark; Nettle root; Oregano; Sal palmetto and Echinacea root are all beneficial.

Option 2: Crateva religiosa and horse tail--soothes the bladder lining and it acts as a diuretic to help relieve spasms.

Option3: A product called "bladder control tea" is beneficial for people who are incontinent. The product is made by Bell Lifestyle Products Inc. And should br available in health stores.

Blemishes-Use benzoyl peroxide which will dry the skin. Afterward, apply tea tree oil, which is an antiseptic and it is antifungal. Green tea or a multi herbal tea may help to reverse damage caused by oxidation. Black willow bark extract is also known to help with skin renewal, while it also works to smooth wrinkles. Aloe Vera gel is also helpful by working to restore UV damage to the skin. Detoxification becomes the first line of defense in the struggle against blemishes because the blemish could be a signal from the body indicating excessive amounts of toxins in the liver.

Cirrohosis –Selenium; milk thistle; lipoic acid (take as directed). Also, a tea composed of steep red oak bark and bay leaves, is helpful. Drink several cups per day. Other herbal teas can also be helpful.

→Detoxification with herbal tea and lavender oil--one drop daily for two weeks and afterward, 1 drop twice a week.

→Take ionic or Colloidal Minerals as directed on label.

→ Take a multi-vitamin.

→Eat cilantro daily for 1 week to detox mercury.

→Take high doses of Vitamin C- a.m. and p.m., however if diarrhea occurs, reduce the amount by one-half.

→Take Vitamin A, three times per day.

→Take Vitamin B-complex pill (maximum potency).

→Take folic acid.

→Take Omega-3 and flax seed oil.

→Lipoic acid–helps to stimulate the liver to produce new cells.

Herbs to take:

→Milk Thistle -protects liver with a defensive coating. Take as directed.

→Turmeric -High in antioxidants.

→Parsley -eat a large amount.

→Hemp Acrimony -take as directed.

→Raw fruit and vegetables -eat a large amount daily.

→Yogurt -take two tablespoons before each meal to receive digestion enzymes.

Also, refrain from eating meat, white flour, white sugar, fried foods. Eat as much raw food as possible or lightly cooked food to get the enzymes necessary for organ rebuilding.

→**Cysts**–potassium iodine–rub on the cyst three times per day.

Cancer--Cancer starts from mutated cells that grow uncontrollably. This growth may be pre-programmed by genetics. Under certain circumstances, something triggers cells to mutate. Examples of what can trigger the change include stress, injury, enzyme tolerances and or a person's diet. Assuming your genetics have predisposed you to cancer, or if you already have cancer, or if you want to try to avoid getting cancer, the following information might be helpful to explore.

Cancer is the second leading cause of death in the United States. It comes in a variety of names, including: breast cancer prostate cancer, lymphomas, colon cancer, pancreatic cancer. It is believed by many that an individual can control his or her destiny by maintaining a proper well balanced diet, along with trying to eliminate stress and by avoiding environmental toxins. This theory is also a good recipe for those people who have or have recovered from some form of cancer. Defense, with regard to cancer, is the best offense.

→**Step 1**–Getting the body's blood alkaline is a must for proper nutrient absorption and a plentiful supply of oxygen for the blood. It also provides an unfriendly environment for pathogens (cancer cells). On the other hand, acidic blood is low in oxygen , poor in nutrients and it is a breeding ground for pathogens (viruses and bacteria). Alkalinity is about minimizing stress because stress is acidic, maximizing raw fruits and vegetables taking supplements and eliminating or reducing meat, dairy products, fried foods, over-processed foods, over-cooked foods (kills the enzymes), alcohol, smoking, white sugar, white flour products, white rice and including more herbs in the diet.

Step 2- This step focuses on eliminating internal toxins within the body; however, the process of keeping them out of the body varies from person to person and depends highly on a person's physical condition. There are various methods (see Chapter Two) and some are more taxing on a person, which ties in with your present condition of health.

Toxins, can be in the form of metals such as mercury (found in fish) aluminum (antiperspirant deodorant), asbestos and petroleum products. They are also found in the air (fumes). Toxins from some foods include, nitrates, antibiotics hormones etc. The list is endless. Nonetheless, the samples provided will give you a better understanding of the problem with toxins in the body.

Toxins enter the blood in various ways, including breathing, drinking and eating; however, the toxins can also enter the body through items such as: cosmetics, insecticides (bug spray), grease and suntan lotion. It is important to remember that if a product is man-made, rather than natural, it is more probable that the item contains ingredients that are incompatible with the body.

Once toxins enter the blood system, they frequently lodge in the body's cells, especially fat, and once entrenched there, they can cause additional problems. A good well-balanced diet, along with drinking lots of water and the use of herbs is a mild approach to detoxification and more importantly the burden on the liver will be lessened.

→**Step 3**-A healthy and nutritional diet is essential. However, supplements are also necessary due to the lack of the necessary nutrition from modern-day food. Organic food is best, but it is important to eat good fats, such as olive oil, butter and nuts; rather than bad oils such as vegetable oils and margarine.

Step 3 has a precondition, which is your digestive tract, which must be in good operating order to properly process the food into nutrients. This means good bacteria must be in place in the stomach and in the intestinal tract. This process includes taking digestive enzymes, eating yogurt or sauerkraut before meals, as they each contain good bacteria. Vinegar also helps stomach acid to properly dissolve the food. Vinegar also helps to keep the body alkaline.

Step 4- As mentioned earlier in step 3, 100 percent of the proper nutrition cannot be obtained from food; therefore it is recommended that you consider the following suggestions:

Eat as much raw food as possible to get the necessary enzymes and nutrients required to strengthen the body's cells and killer T-cells. Organic and free range food should be eaten as often as possible. The proper or key word should be live food, rather than overcooked (dead) food. If you are suffering from cancer, you will want to eat more live food and protein, which can be obtained from beans, fish, poultry and lean meat; however, it is much healthier to refrain from eating all meat, because meat is acidic to the blood.

Glutathione-an antioxidant produced by the body may be in short supply due to cancer so you must supplement your diet or eat food that is high in Glutathione, such as asparagus, avocados, cabbage, walnuts and broccoli.

Vitamin C-an antioxidant that the body needs in large amounts and can be acquired by supplements or by eating lots of vegetables and fruit. Nevertheless, be cautious of eating too much fruit because of its high sugar content, which could become a problem for you if you are borderline diabetic.

Fiber-is good for digestion and it gets rid of excess cholesterol. Foods that are high in fiber include grapes, vegetables, sweet potatoes, yams, brown rice and popcorn.

→Vitamin D3 –a powerful vitamin that may prevent cancer problems. Good food for the liver include onions and garlic, both of which help to detoxify the liver. Garlic contains 80 sulphur compounds, helps purify the blood and it acts as an antiseptic to the body. Multi herbal tea is good for the nutrition contained in the various teas, including green tea, juniper tea (breaks down toxin in fat), lavender tea (good for detoxification), wheat grass, burdock root and milk thistle. It is also helpful to take a high potency multivitamin. Colloidal Minerals offer similar benefits.

Fish oil and flax seed oil- each contain Omega 3-- They improve the immune system.

Chinese mushroom maitake–The mushroom is thought to activate cancer-killing cells.

Milk thistle–a supplement that protects the liver and aids in detoxification.

Herbs-turmeric, fennel seed, cats claw, rosemary, cayenne pepper, Paul d Arco, wormwood and echinacea, each of which are all good for the immune system and they contain anti-cancer properties.

Lysine (Amino acid supplement) combined with high doses of Vitamin C, E and Beta-carnitine supports healthy cell membranes to hinder cancer cells' devastation.

Cancer, Pancreatic--Before any cancer can be beaten, the body and blood must be alkaline. Alkaline blood is not a friendly environment for cancer cells. If you have cancer you probably are acidic, since alkaline people do not get cancer. Stay away from acid causing foods. Red meat, sugar, white flour products, fast food, and processed foods. Eat raw fruit (cancer cells love sugar) and vegetables; however, not too much fruit, because fruit contains natural sugar and cancer cells love sugar.

To regain alkalinity take one tablespoon of apple cider vinegar with water before each meal; eat lots of raw vegetables. Always eat raw fruit on an empty stomach so it doesn't mix with protein and ferment. Eat onions, and lots of raw garlic. The garlic acts as a blood purifier. Also, eat beets, celery and cloves. The clove is an anti cancer fighter, but must be sucked on in the mouth like a lifesaver and as often as possible throughout the day.

Once the body is alkaline, continue the same regimen, but add the following: Anti cancer herbal tea (a detoxification tea, which is also anti- cancer); Ionic minerals; Magnesium tablets; high potency male multi vitamin; zinc and organic cottage cheese, mixed with flax seed oil, with a little cayenne pepper added for good enzymes; fish oil (high quality brand such as Nordic. Take as directed on label; Multi herbal tea; eating yogurt at least twice daily is known to aid in digestion and in nutrient assimilation; Curcumin (contains an anti-cancer ingredient, the herb turmeric); Vitamin C (high doses, however, if you get diarrhea take lower doses.

The following are also helpful in the fight against cancer: Shitake mushrooms–Take as directed; however, it is important that you take a sufficient amount in proportion to your body weight. It is usually recommended that the dosage should be taken on an empty stomach several times a day. It is known to be a good cancer fighter. Wormwood capsules (take as directed) as a cancer-fighting herb used for generations by tribal people.

Hydrazine sulfate capsule--It inhibits the production of glucose from lactic acid in the liver, which will starve the rapidly growing cancer cells. It is very important to use this. Once the tumor begins to shrink, you should notice an increase in the appetite, along with a reduction of pain and some improvement in the person's mood. Simultaneously, blood circulation should improve. Take according to directions.

CoQ10–The body makes CoQ10, but adding the supplement (CoQ10) will increase tissue detoxification and aid in cellular energy. It is imperative that people who take statins also use the supplement because statins prevent the body from making CoQ10. Take as directed on label.

Carpal Tunnel—Caused by a mineral and vitamin deficiency, particularly Vitamin B complex. The herb turmeric helps to relieve inflamation. Other options include multi-herbal teas, including a combination ginkgo biloba, horse chestnut and St. John's wort.

Cholesterol (High)–Chinese red yeast, Niacin (Vitamin B-3) and Policosanol (natural extract from sugar cane), used in combination, is often recommended by physicians to help reduce high cholesterol. This combination is a natural alternative to statins.

1--Getting rid of artery plaque--use lecithin to help dissolve hardened artery plaque in the blood vessels. Some lecithin is contained in cholesterol, however, not in sufficient amounts to singularly remove plaque. Lecithin acts as a drain cleaner of the blood vessels. Zinc works to open up the arteries and CoQ10 utilizes fat to generate energy, while working to help keep arteries clear.

2–A diet that totally excludes meat and or dairy products, including eggs is known to be responsible for more deaths, not less. If you refrain from eating meat and dairy products, you are simultaneously preventing your body from receiving good fats and protein. The standard total rate for cholesterol was 250; but in recent times, the rate has been reduced to 200. The drastic change has affected the lives of a large number of elderly people who have become acclimated to the lower standard, which is causing some to become more susceptible to heart failure because of switching to low cholesterol and or low fat diets.

Need soluble fiber-use fresh ground flax seeds to help oil bond to bile in the intestines and it prevents absorption of cholesterol by the blood. Raw oatmeal (unheated) produces the same effects. Cocoanut oil raises the total cholesterol level, only because HDL goes up and the large amount of fiber in the cocoanut oil reduces LDL levels. Two kinds of carbohydrates, starch-and-sugar and secondly. non-digestible (fiber)–grains, fruits, vegetables consumption, stops cholesterol from oxidating, which occurs when cholesterol causes a problem in artery health. For example, leave an orange slice on the table and watch it change colors. That is caused when the oxygen begins to degrade the fruit; however, when the orange slice is coated with lemon before it is placed on the table, the oxidation process is slowed down. This is why when you make a fruit salad, adding lemon prolongs the time that the salad can be kept in the refrigerator.

Since cholesterol does not dissolve in water, the liver provides fatty acid to attach to the cholesterol and surrounds both with a protein hence the word lipoprotein HDL (high density lipoprotein) and LDL. Both lipoproteins transport to the liver for elimination from the body. The HDL are larger particles that move quickly through the blood; however, the LDL are smaller particles are also sticky, which causes them to cling to artery walls while they travel. These actually lead to ulcers that cause the body to react by forming a clot. Supplementing your diet with fatty acids (Omega 3), which are useful in the production of cell membranes and in the regulating of blood pressure. Omega 3 also helps to lower LDL and it is anti-clotting, anti-inflammatory and food for the brain, which contains 20% fatty acid.

The word cholesterol standing on its own is meaningless unless you know the levels of the HDL, LDL and triglyceride. If the LDL level is 100 or lower, your count is good and HDL high levels do not become a concern. Conversely, low cholesterol usually means nothing; however, if your LDL level is high and your HDL is low, you could be susceptible to having a heart attack. More elderly people suffer heart attacks when their cholesterol levels are low because the HDL is low and the LDL is higher in proportion. The key word is ratio HDL to LDL (low density lipoproteins) and VLDL (very low density lipoproteins). See chart on cholesterol levels below.

Cholesterol Supplements–

→Garlic-three cloves raw daily.

→Artichoke-blocks absorption of cholesterol and they assist the liver in the detoxification of toxic chemicals.

→Psyllium Seed (powder form)-reduces cholesterol and triglycerides. It also prevents the absorption of cholesterol by the body. Take as directed with water. It also helps to prevent constipation.
→Vitamin D-3--naturally from the sun, which is the most effective or it can be taken in supplement form.
→Multi-herbal teas, which contains nutrients and enzymes.
→Apple cider vinegar.
→Raw fruits and vegetables which contain enzymes that aid in the lowering of cholesterol. Raw fruits and vegetables are also effective in assisting with proper digestion.
→Cayenne pepper used in combination with the herb hawthorn work to dilate blood vessels and to remove excess cholesterol.

Cholesterol normal measuring levels:
Normal range– 110-200–over 200 is bad, but look to compare the LDL to HDL ratio before deciding upon treatment.
HDL Level 29-67–transports large cholesterol particles to various organs, which produce hormones. It also aids in cellular repair.
LDL– 62-100–small particles taken to liver via the blood, but sticky particles attach to blood vessels.
VLDL–a measurement of triglycerides in the blood: 0-40 triglycerides is considered good. Triglycerides-41-100-If your count is in this range, it requires attention. Triglycerides are fats; however once the count moves into the required attention zone, the fats begin to reduce the oxygen in the blood, which causes the blood to thicken.

Cholesterol High--A natural combination of supplements that one of my clients received from his M. D. that succeeded in reducing bad cholesterol: Red yeast, Beta Sitosterol and Niacinamide (Vitamin B3). These three reduce the body's absorption of cholesterol; however, it is important to remember that it is the LDL that needs to be reduced, not the HDL which is part of the total cholesterol. You need good HDL to prevent heart disease. Also, good dental hygiene and flossing your teeth regularly, helps to prevent bad bacteria from accumulating in your mouth. In addition, both practices lowers the risk of getting heart disease. Poor dental hygiene can increase C-reactive protein in the blood, which is an indicator of heart disease.

Overweight people usually have high levels of interleukin 6, high cholesterol and C-reactive protein, all of which are inflammatory. Exercise and weight loss reduces inflammation caused by the previously mentioned items.

Concentration should be focused on the buttocks, leg fat and belly fat. In conjunction, it is also important to reduce bad fats such as omega 6, which is a producer of inflammation. Foods to avoid include: vegetable oil, fried foods, processed foods and grain-fed meat.

Other options include:

→Folic acid--protects against heart damage and it is especially helpful after a heart attack.

→Raw garlic- has 80 sulfuric compounds to keep arteries clear.

→Hawthorne-an herb that strengthens blood vessels while it stimulates the heart. It can also be taken as an herbal tea.

→Fish oil lowers triglycerides.

→Magnesium reduces artery calcification.

→ Nattokinase a soybean product that aids the circulation process and dissolves unwanted plaque deposits.

→Pickled beets contain Vitamin B3, which produces nitric oxide to dilate blood vessels.

→Zinc-aids the immune system.

→CoQ10-good for heart.

→Olive oil-a good fat.

→Bromelain–An herb that reduces inflamation. It is also found in pineapple.

Cold Sores--Selenium, garlic, onions and lysine. Selenium is found in both onions and garlic; however, selenium and lysine (amino acid) supplements can also be purchased at health stores. Also, take cigar tobacco (moistened) and press against the inflamed area. The longer you keep the moistened tobacco against the affected area, the chances of lessening the inflamation increases greatly.

COPD (chronic obstructive pulmonary disease)--Mucus is a common problem with COPD. The over production of mucus blocks the airways and becomes a breeding haven for infections and breathing problems. A new product called the Lung Flute produces sound waves that stimulate the mucus removing ability of the cilia and airways to rid the body of mucus – the cost is about $45 and it does require a prescription. Call 1-888-820-0970 or www.lungflute.com.

A common deficiency among people with COPD is that they have a low level of glutathione and other antioxidants that when at their proper levels can help reverse lung tissue damage. Nonetheless, glutathione is not well absorbed unless inhaled. You can try "reduced glutathione" in capsule form; however, the best use of the glutathione is when taken by an inhaler; however, for the latter a prescription is required.

Another useful supplement is a potassium and iodine derivative called SSKI, which is known to help break up mucus; however, a prescription is necessary.

Another over-the-counter product is N-Acetyl-cysteine, an herbal supplement that works to reduce inflammation, while it helps to improves lung capacity. Its also an antioxidant and will restore glutathione levels to fight respiratory malfunctions.

Cracked skin behind ears–Need zinc and essential fatty acids (sunflower seeds, fish oil, pumpkin seeds).

Cracked lips–Dehydration causes chapping, but if the lips are cracked in the corners, the body might be deficient in riboflavin, Vitamin B-12 and the other B Vitamins known as B-complex. If the lips are chapped, it is recommended that you replenish the body by drinking plenty of water; rather than reaching for lip balm. Chapped lips is a direct sign that the body lacks a proper amount of water.

Cramps–The herbs slippery elm, lobelia (contains 14 flavonoids) and Fennel seed powder when added to food helps to ease cramps and eliminate gas.

Crohn's Disease-non-existent in the United States until the 1950s, which was the same time that refined and chemically treated food became available. The disease is thought by some to be caused from food allergies, stress, a deficiency of good bacteria or from a virus. The elimination of processed foods and better eating habits help to alleviate the disease.

Additionally, you should eat organic foods and plenty of protein. Soups and juices help to retain fluid and they are easily digested. They also provide good nutrients to the body. However, you should eliminate beans, cabbage, fried foods, white flour, dairy products, red meat, popcorn, seeds, soda, white rice, sugar, and high fiber foods that may aggravate the bowels. In addition, you should eliminate complex carbohydrates because of the difficulty in digesting such foods and equally alarming, complex carbohydrates produce a source of food for bad bacteria.

Good digestion requires good bacteria. Eat yogurt, digestive enzymes, raw fruit and vegetables. One tablespoon of raw unheated sauerkraut before each meal also delivers needed bacteria to the stomach and its intestinal tract. In conjunction, yogurt does the same thing as raw sauerkraut.

The first order of business is to clean out the digestive system with a three-day fast which should include cabbage juice. Afterward, try the following:

→Aloe vera-take as directed on label. It helps to soothe the digestive tract.

→Fish oil-It helps stop a reccurrence of diarrhea.

→Digestive enzymes-take with each meal.

→Glutamine-This amino acid is food for healthy cells that line the digestive tract. Take before each meal as directed.

→Probiotic such as lactobacillus and acidolphilis-bifidus should be taken as directed on label. Supplies helpful bacteria to digestive tract.
→DGL licorice-Take as directed before meals.
→High potency multivitamin, Colloidal Minerals.

Chest pain–Shortness of breath–Is an indication of a cardiovascular/heart problem. The following supplements are helpful:
→**Coenzyme Q10**; D-Ribose; Carnitine. Each helps to transform fat into energy, while it helps the heart to pump blood; Fish oil; magnesium and Vitamin C. Magnesium is a natural calcium channel blocker, which works to relax the arteries, reduce blood pressure and keeps the calcium in a liquid state in the blood. In conjunction, it is important that the diet contains high amounts of fruits and vegetables because of the antioxidants and enzymes contained in those foods. Also, eating raw vegetables is more beneficial than cooked vegetables.

Canker Sores--usually related to food allergies. Take probiotics such as lactobacillius acidophilus to lessen recurrences. It is also helpful to take Vitamin B-12 sublingually. In addition, the product "Cankermelts" a medicated disc, which is available over the counter and online is also helpful against Canker sores. Also do not use toothpaste that contains sodium lauryl sulphate (SELS).

Celiac disease (commonly referred to as Sprue)-The lack of villi in the small intestines inhibits the absorption of nutrients due to a severe allergy to wheat and gluten, the latter found in wheat products. The disease was not widely known for many years; however, it is primarily known as a Mediterranean disease because the majority of people who are victimized by it are from that region of the world. Long ago, the disease became known during a famine in Europe. Due to the scarcity of wheat, rice was used as a substitute. Afterward, the medical field discovered that after the diets were switched to rice, people suffering with Sprue began getting better.

To this day, the only medical treatment known is a gluten-free diet. Recently, as the mysterious disease has come out of obscurity, you can now usually find foods with labels that are emblazoned with the words "Gluten-free." One side effect of Celiac disease is poor assimilation of nutrients, such as fat soluble Vitamins, A, E, K and D, B-12, calcium, folic acid and iron. The poor assimilation can lead to other diseases. Symptoms can include the following: bloating, irritable bowels, cramps, diarrhea and severe stomach pains. A person who suffers from the disease and breaks the diet by consuming even a tiny piece of wheat can suffer immensely.

→**Cataracts**–caused by too much sugar in the diet. The excess sugar attaches itself to proteins in a process called glycosylation.

→Product called "Nu Eyes"which contains an antioxidant (N-acetylcornosine), which dissolves the cataract. The product is sold as a moisturizer. Use as directed on label. Also, the lens in the eye becomes covered with a film. Take "Nu Eyes." If the cataracts are removed surgically, it can result in far-sightedness. If you have difficulty finding "Nu Eyes," which is an imported product, you can substitute it with another, product "Brite Eyes," which is similar.

→**Chelation**-Use bentonite clay-two tablespoons mixed with eight ounces of water or use in the bath to pull toxins out of pores; use four cups and remain in the bath tub for twenty minutes- has high PH and good absorption for toxins pharmaceuticals and pesticides.

Colds-Option 1-Take Vitamin C tablets and dissolve them with zinc tablets in a little water. Use as a gargle and after you gargle, swallow the mixture. Repeat often. To increase the potency, add some cayenne pepper to the mix.

Option 2- Gargle a little cayenne pepper with honey in tea to kill germs.

Option 3-Echinacea herb does not prevent cold, but it does shorten the duration and severity (1) Herbal Health Watch Michael Castleman Herb Quarterly Magazine.

Option 4–A combination of horse radish, cayenne pepper, garlic and ginger root.

Colds, Coughs and Flu–Take Elencampame, a herb known as the "lung healer"-use the root for tea. It heals the body by driving open the pores which causes the body to sweat. Contains terpenoids and sesquiterpenes and protects the liver.

Colitis– The herb curcumin reduces symptoms or frequency of flare ups. The trick is to keep the bowel clean (detoxification). Take dietary charcoal to absorb toxins-will be excreted by the body with normal body wastes-afterward take aloe to help keep the intestines slippery. Indigestible charcoal absorbs toxins in the intestines. Also, eating too much red meat can aggravate the intestines. Drinking large amounts of red shank tea and taking the supplement selenium in high doses helps to curtail colitis.

Congestive Heart Failure (heart's inability to pump due to fluid buildup)-Take Hawthorne extract, Vitamin E and a diuretic, such as coffee, herbal tea, parsley and watermelon to get rid of excess fluid.

Constipation–Olive oil, papaya, spinach and walnuts help to lubricate the intestines. Other items that are helpful include:

Castor Oil

Coffee, a natural detoxifier also helps to fight constipation.

Fiber rich whole grain bread- works as well as a laxative.

→**Flaxseed oil**, take as directed before each meal; Cascara Sagrada, liquid or capsule. Take daily as directed.

→**Fleet enema**–can be purchased over the counter.

→**Vinegar**-take a small amount of Bragg's Apple Cider Vinegar, mixed with water and honey, in a juice glass.

CVI- A Collection of fluid in the tissue, known also as chronic venous insufficiency, which prevents the blood from getting back to the heart. The impediment causes swelling, cramps and tingles. The cause of this problem is due to a blockage or problems (varicose veins) in the veins. It is recommended that you eat raw garlic, the herb Hawthorne, ginkgo-biloba, Vitamin A, Vitamin D, celery, Colloidal Minerals, calcium and magnesium. It is thought by some that CVI is caused by a breakdown of scavenger cells (Lysosomes). When inactive, these scavenger cells permit fluid to buildup in the lungs.

Depression--Choline, an amino acid, improves nerve impulses. Tryptophan, an amino acid, found in milk turkey and eggs.--take as directed on an empty stomach before bed, because the proteins in the stomach inhibit absorption if taken with meals. Other herbs that are helpful include, St. Johns wort and saffron (substitute for Prozac).

Diabetic Neuropathy--alpha lipoic acid helps regenerate nerves; L-Arginine (nitric acid) aids in circulation, while it protects the artery walls and helps to dilate blood vessels.

Evening primrose oil and fish oil–may help to preserve nerve endings. Take daily as directed.

Gingko biloba- good for circulation, especially in the blood supply to nerve endings.

GLA (gamma linolenic acid)--Borage oil or Black Currant oil, both a source of GLA, are sometimes effective in helping to repair nerve damage, which is known to occur in diabetics who begin to lose the feeling in their feet. Borage oil can be used in combination with Niacinamide (Vitamin B-3), which may aid in the process of helping the pancreas produce insulin. Niacinamide may help to restore pancreas function.

Alpha lipoic acid helps the beta cells in the pancreas and may also be effective in repairing damaged nerves. Grape seed extract, which contains flavonoids, works to protect the blood vessels, eyes, fingers, kidneys and the tips of toes. Another option is Anodyne Therapy (60 UV lights) is known to help repair nerve damaged.

Diabetes 1–When the pancreas is unable to create sufficient insulin. Symptoms include an increase in appetite, weight loss, constant thirst and frequent urination (to get rid of excess sugar). Urine is clear and foamy due to sugar content. Blood sugar range will be over 350. Normal is 80-110. High blood sugar due to low or no insulin output can be life threatening and it can be attributed to other problems including high blood pressure, poor circulation, numbness of feet, fatigue and poor cognitive function (relating to judgment, memory, perception and reasoning). There is no cure for a poor functioning pancreas although there are some herbs and supplements that may help to control blood sugar and reduce the amount of insulin that is produced by the pancreas. These herbs and supplements include bitterguard, bilbury, chromium, fenugreek, gymnema sylvestre, selenium, Vitamin B complex and Vitamin C.

The object is to keep insulin needs as low as possible by maintaining blood sugar below 80-120 mg/dl, while still maintain a diet necessary for nutrition so that cell growth and repair are maintained.

Everything you eat has a carbohydrate count. Some low and some high. Avoid the high and purchase a carbohydrate guide to assist you in determining what you eat.

Exercise is important, as it aids in digestion and enhances the immune system with the assimilation of nutrients. It also lowers blood sugar. The amount of exercise determines the carbohydrates you will need, so do not over exercise unless you know what to eat in carbohydrates so you don't get hyperglycemic. Also don't eat to get full; rather only for energy.

Weight loss is critical since excess weight often times was the precursor for this disease. Incorporate high fiber in the diet to clear out excess cholesterol and is a good source of carbohydrates as opposed to sugar items which catapults your insulin needs. Also when consuming carbs also simultaneously consume protein and low fat, like olive oil or canola oil. Fat and protein slow the carbohydrates' transition time to sugar. Also, fat is a preferred energy source for the cells.

Keep sodium use low as it makes the blood denser and drives up blood pressure. There is enough sodium in food without adding more, but if you cut back on salt, you may want to add foods, rich in iodine to your diet.

Confine alcohol usage to vodka –no carbohydrates.

Keep hydrated – helps cells to detox and circulates nutrition.

Eat smaller meals more frequently to maintain blood sugar.

A balanced diet is 1/3 carbs 1/3 protein and 1/3 fat (low fat).

Diabetes II–occurs when cell receptors become insulin resistant Diabetes II is the more common version of the disease. Symptoms include over weight, high cholesterol, low HDL, high LDL, triglycerides, high blood pressure, fatigue. Also, your blood sugar range of 150-300 should be 80-100. Insulin resistant cells are what Diabetes II is all about, however unlike Diabetes 1, Diabetes II, is curable through diet exercise and a dedicated plan to lose weight. Fifty percent of obese people are insulin resistant; however, most are unaware of the condition because excess carbohydrates are stored as triglycerides in fat.

Understanding Diabetes II is paramount to combating the disease. Sugar in the blood needs a home. The pancreas excretes insulin to escort this sugar (cell energy) to the cells for consumption, but due to the over use of sugar through the years, the cells no longer accept insulin. Consequently the sugar and insulin have no where to go, which creates a whole list of problems, including weight gain, poor circulation, high blood pressure and a lack of energy.

The goal is to reduce the amount of sugar in the blood, reducing the need for insulin production. It sounds easy and it can be if you count calories. Fourteen hundred calories a day is a good goal. In order to combat this disease the body must be in a fighting mode to enable it to defend against both types of diabetes.

Diabetes 1 and II, uses the following guidelines:

PH levels must be alkaline. This will not only improve the immune system to protect it from viruses and bacteria but it will also help reduce insulin needs. Good PH needs good digestion. This is a must for proper carbohydrate metabolism and nutrient assimilation Also, diabetics are normally deficient in chromium, magnesium, vanadium (trace minerals), zinc, Vitamin B-6 and Vitamin C.

Good digestion requires stomach bacteria and enzymes along with a good supply of hydrochloric acid. All are produced in the stomach, however, the stomach usually requires help through additional digestive enzymes contained in apple cider vinegar. They help bolster the hydrochloric acid which is produced in the stomach when a person eats. In addition to apple cider vinegar, a small portion of yogurt and or raw unheated sauerkraut also provides good stomach bacteria before eating a meal.

Good digestive enzymes metabolize fat and oils, which is helpful to the pancreas, which otherwise would find the fats and oils very difficult to handle. Keeping blood sugar levels stable is the primary goal because high insulin will increase body weight and restrict circulation, which may bring about high blood pressure. Nonetheless, the body still requires energy, so it becomes equally important that you do not convince yourself that you need low carbohydrates.

Refined carbohydrates should be avoided; however, complex carbohydrates are a good source of energy, fiber, minerals and vitamins. Sources for these complex carbohydrates include: artichokes; asparagus; beans; corn; grains; grapefruit; grapes, mushrooms; oatmeal; peaches; popcorn; potatoes; rice (wild and brown); tomatoes; yams and yogurt. Also, if you do not consume a sufficient amount of good carbohydrates, you may become susceptible to fatigue and your insulin levels will become more difficult to stabilize.

The lack of good carbohydrates will also destabilize your blood sugar. Suggested supplements include: a good multi-vitamin that contains high levels of B-complex (reduces insulin need) especially B-6; magnesium, zinc and Colloidal Minerals (good for the chromium and Vanadium, which is usually deficient in people suffering from diabetes). Chromium and Vanadium are known to reduce sugar cravings and to strengthen cell membranes. They also aid in the production of insulin and they also work to protect the eyes.

Alpha lipoic acid-- helps beta cells in the pancreas and it may help to regenerate damaged nerves.

Berberine–the herb helps cells to become more receptive to insulin.

Fenugreek- lowers blood glucose and it reduces insulin production. It also reduces triglycerides and raises HDL. Fenugreek contains fiber, which slows down the food process in the stomach (turning food into sugar).

Ginkgo biloba--good for circulation especially in blood supply to nerve endings.

GLA (gamalinole acid)--Borage oil, a source of GLA, is sometimes effective in slowing nerve damage, which is known to occur in diabetics who begin to lose feeling in their feet. Borage oil can be used in combination with Niacinamide (Vitamin B-3) which may aid in the process of helping the pancreas produce insulin.

Grape seed extract--full of anthocyanins and proanthocyaanidins both flavonoids protect blood vessels of eyes kidneys tips of toes and fingers.

Gymnema Sylvestre- the most common diabetes herb. Gymnema is a component that acts directly on the tongue to block sweet tastes. It also stimulates the pancreas to produce more insulin.

L-Arginine (nitric acid)--aids in circulation, while it protects the artery walls and helps to dilate blood vessels.

Evening primrose oil --helps support nerve endings.

Diabetics are more susceptible to the adverse effects of diabetes when a person's blood levels are low in calcium or Vitamin D.

Dialysis–For complications due to dialysis--use herbal teas, Colloidal Minerals, vitamins, nutritious food, fruits, vegetables and Vitamin D. It is also important that you exercise regularly.

Cinnamon extract--stimulates the production of glucose (real cinnamon is toxic) burning enzymes. One product that is available over the counter is "CinnaBetic II" helps the cells absorb glucose, while it helps to reduce LDL.

Sugar intake initiates insulin production. Once the insulin handles the sugar, the excess insulin prompts additional cravings for sugar. Sugar substitutes act similarly by generating insulin; however, the substitute lacks sugar, while the tongue expects sugar and signals the pancreas to produce insulin. Consequently, the insulin has no sugar to transport. The lack of the sugar causes the additional cravings, which can create more fat cells and it can cause serious damage to the organs.

Poor circulation is a by-product of diabetes. Garlic improves the blood flow, and works to lower blood pressure, while it reduces bad cholesterol. An over-the-counter product, Kyolic is helpful. Take as directed. Another option is to eat plenty of raw garlic. Another food that is helpful in the fight against high blood pressure and diabetic obesity is beans.

If you suffer from Type 2 Diabetes, which is usually the result of a diet that is high in carbohydrates and low in fiber. It is important that you hold to a proper diet that is high in fiber, low in carbohydrates, contains good fats and proteins. The diet that includes good fats and proteins is an excellent source of energy, more so than carbohydrates. However, diet alone is not sufficient. It is equally important that you exercise consistently. Your diet should include large portions of water to prevent dehydration and should also include supplements such as those listed below:

Fruit, nuts and seeds; multi-grain bread; at least one apple a day; one tablespoon of ground flaxseed three times per day (once with each meal). The flax seed is a good fat.

Alpha Lipoic Acid helps circulation to the peripheral nerves. GLA (gamma linolenic acid) serves the same purpose. Diabetics require much more antioxidants than someone who does not suffer from the disease. The following supplements are helpful: Chromium (Chromium deficiency is linked to diabetes); onions, garlic, wheat germ, cheese, and whole grains should be included in the diet); Cinnamon extract; Coenzyme Q10 (usually low in diabetics); American ginseng before each meal to help control blood sugar; Red Grapes, which contain Phytochemicals that help to protect your vision; Gymnema Sylvestre (improves insulin production in pancreas); Magnesium (good for the eyes); olive oil and lots of fish and fish oils; Purslane extract, an herb which helps to curb the appetite and reduce the glucose metabolism; Red shank tea or Queen of the meadow tea–drink frequently on a daily basis; Trace mineral Vanadyl Sulfate (may help to reverse diabetes and lower blood sugar.

The following vitamins should also be taken:

Vitamin B-3, known also as niacinamide (may help to improve the function of the pancreas). Also, take the herb bilberry, which is helpful for circulation and it is good for the eyes, heart and kidneys. People with diabetes benefit from protein in the diet, because it helps smooth out blood sugar levels. Vitamin B complex, Vitamin C and Vitamin E are also helpful.

It is important that you keep insulin from spiking. You should eliminate candy, soda, and other foods that contain refined sugar. Also, eliminate white bread and cut back on saturated fats, such as those found in red meat and dairy products. It is also important that you do not eat too much fruit because fruit contains natural sugar, which is still sugar.

Diabetes could be referred to as the "excess calorie disease" or lifestyle disease. Also known as Diabetes 1 and 2. Diabetes in the US is the 3rd most frequent disease. The common problem for those who suffer from diabetes is carbohydrates, which are broken down by the body's metabolism for cell energy. Carbohydrates also provide food for good intestinal bacteria and it helps with the communications that pass between various cells. However not all carbohydrates are the same.

Complex carbs (good carbs) and refined carbs (bad carbs) are two categories that diabetics must recognize to control their blood sugar.

Diarrhea–The following foods and herbs are helpful in stopping diarrhea:

Apples (apple skins contain the same ingredient (pectin) as Kaopectate. Pectin is the soluble fiber that binds to the body's waste which is excreted. Another supplement known to be helpful in cleaning the bowels is bentonite clay, which is also a good fiber. Carrots-(cooked carrots prevents e-coli from sticking to the intestines); garlic; grapefruit (fights parasite infections); Oregon grape root and Pepto Bismol (contains the mineral bismuth, which helps to eliminate bad bacteria). Yet other supplements include: red root tea, .cinnamon tea or blackberry root tea. The herbs slippery elm and lobelia are also helpful to the bowels when taken as a tea and they also work to relieve cramps.

Diet– The following foods and supplements can be helpful in the diet if the purpose is to lose weight:

Option 1–The herb chickweed and queen Anne's lace taken before each meal dulls appetite and speeds up metabolism.

Option 2- Dried burdock root–eaten either raw or cooked reduces fat and helps to lower blood sugar.

Option 3-Alfalfa and Kale, which contain high amounts of nutrients, minerals and vitamins, are both helpful in the struggle to lose weight. Option 4- Green Tea –Drink green tea multiple times per day. The tea works to dissolve fat; however, it must be green tea, rather than black tea. In England, the people are known for consuming large amounts of meat and potatoes; however, they also consume equally large amount of tea which helps them to remain thin in spite of their diets.

Option 5- eat garlic and ginger on regular basis.

Option 6- dried burdock root raw or cooked purifies blood reduces fat and regulates blood sugar. Alfalfa and chickweed promotes weight loss.

Option 7– Banana leaf is known to reduce fat, while it helps to build muscle.

Option 8-Taking the mineral chromium, which is usually deficient in diabetics works well in suppressing sugar cravings.

Option 9-The herb Glycyrrhizin Glabra otherwise known as Glyabridin is an antioxidant and flavonoid. It helps to reduce body fat, while it also helps to regulate blood sugar.

Option 10–Fenugreek, an herb that is high in fiber content helps to raise HDL levels, reduce triglycerides and slows down the process by which sugar enters the blood.

Diet (weight loss) Ketosis is one of the body's mechanisms used to extricate energy from body fat. Ketosis can not be initiated by fasting. Fasting essentially creates an illusion. While the person who begins to fast in an effort to lose weight, the actual effect is that the body instead loses muscle mass. Ketosis can be activated by maintaining a brown rice and fruit diet, which will begin to help lower calcium in the blood, while it works to lower protein, fat and sodium. Once the body resorts to Ketosis through the diet, the energy is extracted from the fat. Ketosis becomes an alternative energy source when glucose is exhausted.

Digestion problems--Poor digestion is the primary reason that causes poor nutrient assimilation, which can cause the body to become deficient in vitamins, minerals, and enzymes. Chamomile tea aids in digestion and it prevents acid reflux. Some good sources of food that increase good bacteria and enzymes include yogurt, uncooked sauerkraut, apple cider vinegar, angelica tea. Other sources to aid in digestion are probiotics such as: acidophilus, which are available over the counter.

Diverticulitis--The problem known as diverticulitis is a result of some western diets, which may create pouches in the intestines that become irritated and inflamed. Undigested food, small seeds from fruit and even nuts, can cause the problem, which is much easier to prevent than it is to treat. Diverticulitis is essentially non-existent in high fiber whole wheat food diets. A major cause of diverticulitis is constipation. Consequently, it is important to remain regular to avoid suffering from the disease. To help to avoid diverticulitis, the diet should include soluble fiber such as ground flax seed and or oat bran. The flax seed contains omega 3, which is helpful against the disease.

Digestive enzymes in such food as yogurt should be eaten before each meal. The supplement "lactobacillus acidophilus" an excellent digestive enzyme should be taken (as directed on label). It is also beneficial to eat large portions of raw vegetables, along with eating plenty of olive oil. Vitamin C and vegetable juice should be taken for three consecutive days to clean out the toxins that have built up due to irregular bowel function. Fried foods should be totally eliminated from the diet and red meat consumption should be kept at a minimum. A supplement that may be helpful is peppermint oil in capsule form. The peppermint oil capsules help to reduce gas, while it also helps to reduce cramps.

Dizziness--Causes include poor nutrition, bad eating habits, an iron deficiency and a Vitamin B complex deficiency. There are many other things that can cause dizziness including the following: brain tumors; food allergies; low blood sugar; thyroid (under active); prescription drugs; stress and sinus problems (which can effect the inner ear); anemia (low iron). The most common cause of dizziness is poor nutrition, combined with poor circulation. Another cause of dizziness is poor blood flow to the brain.

The following items are helpful when suffering from dizziness:

Multi vitamin high in iron and separate B complex vitamin (can also be obtained from brewers yeast, brown rice, and raw vegetables); Colloidal Minerals for mineral deficiencies; Ginkgo Biloba (take daily with raw garlic (several cloves) along with a few sticks of celery (per day); the herb Ashwagandha (take as directed); the herbs Hawthorne and Panax ginseng, both of which are also good for circulation.

Adrenal gland problems (due to dizziness)--Weak adrenal glands have side effects. For instance fatigue, salt craving, stomach pain, skin blotches, and joint pain. All this is in response to a low production of glucocorticoids a steroid hormone which regulate glucose metabolism. Synthetically produced glucocorticoids are available if you have adrenal insufficiency. There are minerals, vitamins, and herbs which may also help with adrenal gland support. They include: Hi potency multi vitamin; Colloidal Minerals, calcium with Vitamin D and magnesium; Garlic – a blood purifier; Ginseng – good for the adrenal glands. Ginseng and adrenal glandular tablets also support the immune system. It is also important that you detoxify your body. See Chapter Two on detoxification.

You can take a self-test to determine if the adrenal gland is functioning properly. Lie on your back for a minute or two before rising quickly. If you become light-headed, you require adrenal gland support, which includes a cutback on sugar intake and an increase of eating high protein foods.

Dry Skin–See Skin (Dry).

Dysplasia--(Cervical dysplasia which is the growth of non-cancerous cells that grow on the cervix)--women should take folate everyday for two months. For additional information, see National Cancer Institute website: http://www.cancer.gov/

Detoxify with dandelion root, which balances hormones and stimulates digestive tract. Detox can also be accomplished with Burdock root.

Oregano geranium, an herb that is available in a liquid or dry form can help detox heavy metals and it is a free radical scavenger.

Eczema–The presence of eczema indicates a problem with the immune system and it points to a low intake of fatty acids, as well as a poor diet. In addition it also indicates poor digestion, allergies and chromium mal-absorption. The following should be used to counter the eczema: folic acid cream, which should be applied topically; take Colloidal Minerals also known as trace minerals; ionic minerals (contain chromium); fish oil and flax seed for Omega 3; zinc; herbal tea; dandelion, red clover. Other detoxifying digestive enzymes (probotics), including yogurt, or sauerkraut all have good bacteria that is necessary for digestion and nutrients; take before meals. Also, vinegar (preferably apple cider vinegar)–take a little dose (can be mixed with a glass of water) before each meal to assist the stomach acids to digest the food. The vinegar also works to eliminate heart burn (acid reflux).

Raw fruits and vegetables provide nutrients and enzymes which help in the digestion process. Also green and orange vegetables are high in vitamins. Both types of vegetables are good for the skin.

Avoid all white flour, white sugar, white rice and over-processed foods as they provide little nutrients and can be loaded with preservatives. Eczema can also be allergic reaction to chemicals used in food preparation.

Topical application includes neem oil, calendula (a herb oil), liquid Vitamin C and grape seed extract. Mix in equal amounts to create an effective antioxidant that should be applied topically.

Most people who suffer from eczema find that it is caused by an allergic reaction that originates in the small intestines. Once the small intestines is brought back into order, the eczema will resolve itself. Also, Vitamin B-12 cream can help correct the immune system malfunction that caused the eczema. However, stress can also be a source of skin problems.

Chinese violet tea (root or leaf) fights inflammation and dissolves lumps; use with dandelion, red clover and Oregon grape root as a tea. Skin problems can be linked to the liver's need to detox. Use the herbs milk thistle, turmeric, burdock root and lavender. Carrots are also beneficial. Also, taking a bath or washing with a magnesium solution helps to repair skin cells.

Eczema-Antiperspirants contain drying ingredients such as aluminum sulphate. Consider switching to a natural antiperspirant, some of which contain baking soda. Also, homemade bath oil is helpful: mix ½ cup of castor oil with 12 drops of pine, mint, or rosemary scented oil. Store in a closed jar. Add one teaspoon of the mix to the water each time you bathe. If your eczema is found to be caused by allergies, it may be useful to give yourself a pulse test. If you eat something that triggers an allergic reaction, your puse rate goes up.

Epilepsy (disease of abnormal neurotransmitter function) is not completely controllable, despite the best available medications. In many instances, epilepsy requires a trigger to ignite it. Some examples would be: flashing lights, reading, menstrual cycle, cardiovascular disease, stress and contact with pesticides.

Diet is one way to help control seizures. One diet, which includes high fat low carbohydrates is an old remedy from the 1920s that reemerged about 1990. The time-tested remedy reduces seizures by about one-third. Also, a supplement named DMG and apple cider vinegar increase oxygen levels in the blood to reduce lactic acid accumulations, which could be a trigger leading to a seizure.

Colloidal Minerals are a combination of 74 minerals that are essential for the body to be able to function properly; take as directed. A good multi vitamin, combined with detoxification can also be very helpful, especially if the body toxins are a trigger that causes a seizure. Detoxification should include a drop of lavender mixed into a multi-herbal tea. Take the tea daily for two weeks. Afterward, take it every third day for maintenance.

Another helpful addition to the diet would be the inclusion of enzymes, which are usually deficient in the western world where food is more often than not, over refined and over cooked. The body requires digestive enzymes, which are contained in foods including yogurt and sauerkraut. Enzymes can also be obtained in probotics (store-bought enzymes) and liquid acidophius bifidus, which also help to improve digestion and nutrient assimilation from the food you eat.

Vinegar is also helpful in detox, digestion, body alkalinity and overall health. One tablespoon of vinegar, mixed with water, should be taken before each meal. Apple cider vinegar is the best for you because it gets the enzymes from the apples.

Epilepsy supplements:

High potency Multivitamin-aids in brain function.

Vinpocetine--stops the destruction of the nerves and increases the blood flow throughout the brain–Take as directed. Vinpocetine is called an alkaloid found in the periwinkle plant.

Feverfew- a flower herb used to treat migraines. Take as directed.

Ginkgo Biloba- a bioflavanoid that supports mental health as it increases circulation. Take as directed.

St. John's wort- a herb that keeps the nervous system in high gear due to its ability to lower levels of the enzyme monoamine oxidase, which depletes the brain of norepinephrine, a necessary adrenal gland by product that stimulates the nervous system. Take daily as directed.

Liquid Colloidal Minerals-74 trace minerals which used to be in the soil. Take as directed. Many diseases are related to mineral deficiencies.

Fish oil with EPA/DHA--improves neurotransmitter function.

Low levels of calcium, magnesium and Vitamin D--can cause muscle spasms and nerve related problems.

Detox-Mmetal build up in the blood is toxic. Detox liver with multi-herbal tea and 1 drop of lavender oil daily. Bentonite clay, mixed with water also detoxifies heavy metals.

Erectile dysfunction–Frequently, this problem may be a sign of poor circulation. L-arginine (amino acids) dilates blood vessels. Take as directed on an empty stomach. You may also combine L-arginine with pycnogenol (available at health stores), which is similar to taking Viagra.

Other foods and supplements to combat erectile dysfunction:

→Fresh raspberries dilate blood vessels.

→Fava beans contain L-dopa, which stimulates sex drive.

→Onions, garlic, Fenugreek seed and Asian ginseng also work to stimulate the sex drive.

→Yohimbe- take as directed--Tincture increases sex drive.

→Excess sugar intake may reduce testosterone production.

→Pine bark extract-- a sex stimulator.

→Horny goat weed, Arnica (Arnica montana) or ashwagandha (a herbal Viagra)–sex stimulators.

→Chyawanprash–A fruit product. Take with warm milk or on toast.

→Gokshura seed pod promotes sex and velvet bean contains L-dopa a chemical in the brain that affects the mood and sex drive, while it inhibits the hormone prolactin, which can cause ED.

→Soy beans are full of female hormones--leads to impotence and mental decline. The Chinese only use soy very sparingly as a seasoning; however, there is an exception. The Chinese use soy in large amounts when used as a fertilizer. Soy is found in about 60 % of food items available in stores and supermarkets.

Fibromialgia–The symptoms of Fibromialgia include: chronic pain and fatigue, however the cause remains unknown. There are a large number of theories that center around the causes of this disease, including but not limited to infection, stress, trauma, low seratonin levels and the need to detoxify metals such as lead and mercury, along with toxins.

Suggestions: Detox the body of toxins to clean up the liver.

→Colloidal Minerals for trace mineral support.

→Raw fruits and vegetables contain sulfur compounds and are anti-inflammatory.

→Diet: (1/3 carbohydrate, 1/3 protein, 1/3 fat): relies on the glycogen in fat for energy, rather than insulin.

→Malic acid--reduces fatigue and should be taken as directed before meals. Malic acid is also contained in apples, particularly in the skin. It is also found in lower quantities in other fruits and vegetables.

→Bragg Amino Acid--reduces blood sugar and creates enzymes for the immune system.

→C0Q10--Good for function of the heart. It adds additional oxygen to the blood. C0Q10 is also created by the body.

→Vitamin B3--Good for muscle weakness.

→Magnesium–increases energy and should be taken as directed before meals.

→Multivitamin--especially niacin, which can be taken separately; it is also known as Vitamin B3.

→Multi-herbal Tea–containing lots of herbs, including basil, cayenne pepper, oregano, Rosemary and tumeric.

→Alfalfa tablets – full of nutrients.

→Fish oil and flax seed oil – contains prostaglandins, which is anti-inflammatory. Fish oil also prevents cell oxidation.

→Eat high fiber and eliminate sugar and processed foods.

→**Food poisoning**---lemon mixed with sea salt and honey helps to forestall dehydration in combination with activated charcoal (as directed) to absorb poisons in the digestive track. Bragg's Apple Cider Vinegar also kills bad bacteria.

Gallbladder--Bile is required for digestion of food - carried from the gallbladder which aids in fat digestion. Indigestion due to fats indicates poor gallbladder function.

A lack of bile makes fats indigestible and then excreted in the feces which will be brown in color. The body needs bile salts to emulsify fats. Bile salts also aids in the assimilation of Vitamin A, D, E and K, which are fat soluble and cannot be absorbed without fat. Take as directed before meals. Also drinking a multi herbal tea during meals helps emulsify fats. Oregano Oil can jump start the liver and gallbladder to stimulate bile production.

Gallbladder Problems:

The gallbladder stores bile made by the liver to break down fats, it acts like a detergent to emulsify fats for absorption by the body. Gallbladder problems are caused by poor diet, low fiber, poor digestion, low stomach acid and can lead to poor liver function causing bile to become thicker and crystalize becoming gallstones. When a gallstone moves into the gallbladder bile duct, it can get stuck, causing pain and at times, become infected.

Gallbladder removal can lead to digestive problems due to the lack of fats being broken down for the body's absorption. Other symptoms may occur like stomach pain, bloating, itchy skin, increased allergies, gas and diarrhea, not mention a congested liver and/or liver stones.

Diet needs to be low fat (unfortunately can lead to heart attacks) lots of fiber, drink a lot of fluid. Avoid contaminating the liver by staying away from contaminates.

Stay away from high carbs, hydrogenated oils, white sugar and white flour.

Eat yogurt and sauerkraut for digestive enzymes which will aid in digestion in probiotics before each meal for the rest of your lift to aid in digesting fats especially good fats like Omega 3.

Drink tea, especially herbal teas to help break down fats after or during meals. Exercise also aids in fat digestion and absorption.

Bitter herbs before meals also help activate the bile flow from the liver. Herbs like nettle, horsetail or Chinese bitters will suffice.

Last but not least, the problem with the congested liver should not be taken lightly since it is taking over the work of the gallbladder. Congestion is a real possibility. Suggest every 6 months, detox the liver. This can be done with one (1) drop of organic lavender oil in tea, once a day for 2 weeks. Plus take the herb milk thistle every day for life to provide on-going detox and liver protection.

Gallstones--The liver and the gallbladder work together; however, if the gallstones are created by excess calcium, the problem becomes more serious; therefore, it is important to dissolve the stones as quickly as possible. The following supplements should be helpful: magnesium (dissolves excess calcium); Vitamin C; Vitamin E (scavenges free radicals): Omega 3 controls cholesterol and it helps to digest other fats. Drink one cup of freshly squeezed lemon juice mixed with 1 cup of olive oil. Afterward, lie on your right side for two hours until the stone dissolves or passes. An old time remedy: eat cooked turnips to dissolve or prevent a stone from forming. The Koreans and Chinese use the turnips to make a tea. Bile becomes over saturated with calcium.

The body requires hydrochloric acid (also available in tablets and capsules)to help maintain proper digestion. Nonetheless, if a person lacks the proper amount of hydrochloric acid, gall stones can develop. Take hydrochloric acid, as directed before each meal. Fiber is also necessary to help control excess cholesterol.

The following foods contain fiber: fruit (particularly apples and apple skins); beans and leafy green vegetables. If you have gallstones, milk thistle cleans and works to help repair the liver, while simultaneously working to help reduce cholesterol concentrations. Also, dandelion leaves or root activates bile production to keep the gallbladder from getting saturated with a build-up of calcium and cholesterol. Yet another helpful supplement is peppermint which works to help keep the bile duct lubricated.

Glaucoma- liquid that circulates within the eye for nourishment loses its ability to drain out of the eye ducts. The pressure used to force the liquid back into the veins builds up, causing pressure on the optic nerve. Also, the eye cells light sensitivity becomes impaired.

Some supplements that are helpful include L-Arginine, L-carnitine and high doses of Vitamin C and Vitamin D. An excellent source for Vitamin C can be obtained by eating apples, including the skin. However, other good sources of Vitamin C can also be found in fruits and vegetables. Herbs that are beneficial include rose hips and rutin, both of which strengthen the capillaries in the eyes. Detoxification is also important for those who suffer from glaucoma.

Graves Disease–See Thyroid, Hyperactive.

Gums (bleeding)–A build up of plaque which requires a dental technician's cleaning and supplements with coenzymes Q10 and folate. Take as directed. A folate mouth wash may also be helpful. The following are also beneficial: oregano oil, grape root and sage used as a mouth rinse. You can also use tea tree oil mixed with water as a mouth wash to kill bacteria.

Hair--for shiny healthy hair massage 2 raw eggs into hair and let it sit for about ten minutes before washing.

Dry Hair-–massage your hair with mayonnaise and rinse about once a week.

Oily Hair–Shampoo your hair regularly as usual and afterward, rinse with lemon juice.

Hangovers--Vitamin B complex (includes all of the B Vitamins), which helps to break down the alcohol. Drinking large amounts of water is important because it overcomes dehydration, which was initially caused by the consumption of the alcohol. Drinking Gatorade is also helpful when dealing with a hangover, because it replaces electrolytes lost from consuming the alcohol. Another remedy in use for ages is raw honey and toast. Bragg's Apple Cider Vinegar is also good.

Headaches (Migraine)--Migraines are often caused by allergic reactions to food preservatives like nitrates and other toxins. This can be from work related fumes like cooking oils, hair solutions and cleaning solutions. Actually, nearly everyone is surrounded by toxins, but when they build up in the blood, it can trigger migraines.

Also, some women suffer from migraine headaches following the end of the menstruation cycle due to low estrogen, which causes a drop in the hormone serotonin. During pregnancy, a woman has high estrogen and high serotonin, which is why migraine headaches are usually non-existent during pregnancy. Eating chocolate, spinach, greens, milk or shrimp helps to increase seratonin level. Supplements such as 5-htp, which contains serotonin, are available over the counter. Also, with regard to women, migraines can be caused by a hormonal imbalances.

Another cause of migraines can be attributed to a deficiency in calcium and magnesium. This deficiency can be caused by drinking carbonated soda, which is known to deplete the body of calcium and magnesium.

A magnesium deficiency can be the result of using antacids and birth control pills. The first step in combating migraine headaches is to detoxify the body (see Chapter Two on detoxification). The next step is to put your digestive tract in order by modifying your diet by eating more raw foods and foods that contain good digestive enzymes such as yogurt and sauerkraut. Digestive enzymes are also available over the counter.

It is also important that your diet includes fiber, which can be acquired by eating fruits and vegetables. Drinking plenty of water, which aids in detoxification, also helps in preventing dehydration and constipation. In the event that you suffer from heartburn, it may be helpful to drink a little bit of vinegar before eating. The vinegar helps the food to digest by supplying acid to the stomach. You can also take hydrochloric acid tablets, which are available at health food stores.

Once your system is detoxified and the digestive tract is providing nutrition, make sure the nutrition does not include a lot of red meat, fried foods, over cooked food, processed food or dairy products. Eat as much raw or lightly cooked food as possible. If the food is cooked well-done, the process will kill the food enzymes, which are necessary (enzymes) for the body, because they are the catalyst that permits the cells to function properly.

The above mentioned supplements are essential because many nutrients are no longer acquired through the foods we eat (over-farmed and processed foods). Consequently, due to the lack of proper nutrients, supplements become necessary to compensate for the deficiency. These include: multivitamins; Colloidal Minerals; Coenzyme Q10 (good for circulation); alpha lipoic acid, which helps cells regenerate and magnesium (needed for calcium absorption and cellular repair).

In addition to the above, the herb butterbur plant is also known to be effective against migraines; take as directed. Other helpful supplements include: Vitamin B2 and magnesium.

Heart Disease--A wide approach is needed to help cover a multitude of heart problems. The answer starts with diet, which should include more fiber (soluble) from fruit, vegetables and grain. Whole grain bread and beans are recommended. Fats are part of your cell structure. Good fats, like those from coconut oil, fish, olive oil, and even butter fit the menu. Antioxidants, including herbs like cayenne, garlic, green teas, herbal teas and turmeric also help the immune system.

What to avoid–refined carbohydrates and sugar because with both (refined carbohydrates and sugar), the excess turns into triglycerides. Avoid eating large amounts of saturated fat from meat and dairy products. Moderation is the key. Also avoid trans fats from fried and processed foods.

Drinking wine and eating red grapes and cherries, can help to lower cholesterol in the blood. Tea is helpful because it acts as a detergent that helps break up fatty acids. Cholesterol will be less of a problem if you adhere to the above diet. However, other minor items can also help and these include taking bitter herbs. The herbs work to prompt the liver to activate the gallbladder, which then passes bile into the intestines and from there it is excreted. In conjunction, the process works to prevent the intestines from reabsorbing toxins, bile and cholesterol.

The following items, including particular foods and herbs that are helpful in maintaining a healthy heart, are: drinking one alcoholic beverage per day, which will dilate the blood vessels; eat several garlic cloves each day; Ginkgo biloba, take as directed; Hawthorne, take as directed; Ginger; Alfalfa and Bilberry. The herb Bilberry which works similarly to spinach, helps to strengthen the walls of the arteries; Siberian ginseng, take as directed. Mothers wart and Niacin (Vitamin B3) are also helpful in lowering cholesterol.

Heart Disease can also be the result of the calcification of the arteries, which can be the result of too little or too much calcium. Too much calcium, results in the excess calcium collecting inside the arteries. It is possible that taking too many calcium supplements is the cause. Calcium can be a two-edged sword, which makes it extremely important that the proper calcium levels be maintained.

However, too little calcium in the blood may cause the body to initiate a defensive mechanism that works to remove calcium from the bones. The body then floods the blood with calcium to keep the blood alkaline, and in turn the calcium feeds the cells and nerves. This flow of excess calcium begins to collect in the arteries and joints, which may lead to other problems, including kidney stones. Nevertheless, even a blood test can be deceiving by falsely indicating good calcium levels, after the calcium had literally permeated the blood.

If you have low calcium levels, the following supplements may be helpful: boron, copper, magnesium, strontium, and Vitamin D. In conjunction, the previously mentioned minerals are all contained in Colloidal Minerals.

Heartburn: Is usually caused by not having sufficient acid in the stomach.

Option 1–take one tablespoon of vinegar, mixed with water before meals.

Option 2–drink chamomile tea to help prevent heartburn.

Option 3–take DGL tablets as directed.

Heel spurs can be caused by a lack of calcium in the diet due to poor circulation. Poor digestion can also be caused by a lack of Vitamin K2, minerals, magnesium, copper, boron and Vitamin D.

Hemorrhoids–apply petroleum jelly and zinc oxide as needed. You can also use rutin (known also as quercetin, which is available over the counter. Use it externally along with liquid Vitamin C cream to help strengthen the walls of the blood vessels. Another supplement, olive oil, is also helpful. It should be eaten at each meal to help keep the bowels lubricated. Castor Oil applied to anus is also helpful.

Hemochromatosis – (too much iron in the blood) – The first line of defense is a good immune system and the next phase is to take the supplements or follow along with the immune building recommendation. It is important that you prevent iron, which becomes toxic, from accumulating in the body, particularly the joints and organs. Too much iron in the body can also contribute to causing various illnesses, including Alzheimer's disease, arthritis, diabetes, Parkinson's disease and even impotence.

→Colloidal Minerals (contains 74 trace minerals)- Take at bedtime.

→Multi herbal tea with 1 drop of lavender daily. This is for the detoxification of the liver and it also supports the immune system.

→Multi Vitamin

→Milk Thistle – to protect the liver. Taken as directed.

→Prolysinc–Take as directed to help build cell collagen.

→Vitamin B-6 – helps build red blood cells and helps the nerves and muscles to function; take as directed.

→Metal magnet –An over-the-counter product that helps to remove heavy metals from your body.

→Cell power – a supplement to help keep body alkaline by enhancing cell health. Take as directed.

Hepatitis C–it is helpful to take selenium; milk thistle and lipoic acid; take as directed. Lipoic acid is helpful in promoting new cell life and it also works to suppress the increase of hepatitis cells. Other supplements that are helpful against Hepatitis C include: Colloidal Minerals, multi vitamin; alpha lipoic acid and selenium (antiviral). Another useful supplement is the herb silymarian. The above mentioned supplements all help to prevent or lessen inflammation. Also eat raw foods as often as possible. They retain many of the enzymes that are lost during the cooking process. Yogurt and sauerkraut are also known to be helpful to the digestive system.

It is also very helpful if you use alcoholic beverages moderately. Alcohol consumption should be limited to red wine. Heavy drinking of alcoholic beverages is known to impede the detoxification process by reducing the glutathione level in the liver, which hinders the glutathione from assisting in the process. A reduction in glutathione, which works to block triglycerides from building in the liver, can also lead to cirrhosis of the liver.

Supplement your diet with glutathione and eat foods that are rich in glutathione. These foods include: asparagus, broccoli, brussels sprouts, cabbage, cauliflower, kale and spinach. Herbs that are helpful include: turmeric, Omega 3 and niacin (Vitamin B3), which helps (similarly to glutathione) to block triglycerides from forming in the liver. Yet another helpful supplement to combat Hepatitis C, is thymus extract.

Hives–Could be caused by an allergic reaction or stress. Hives can also be the result of poor digestion caused by low levels of stomach acid.

Hormone Imbalance–Hormone imbalance is caused by too little of some hormones and not enough of others. The production of hormones is the job of the endocrine system that includes glands like the pituitary, thymus, thyroid, adrenal, pancreas, testes and the ovaries. Some hormones, such as prolactin for women, flow in the blood stream and aids in the production of breast milk. Other examples include Andrenocorticotrophin, a thyroid hormone that regulates fat. Yet another example is somatotrophin, a growth hormone that works to regenerate cells and bones. Somatotrophin also works to produce estrogen, progesterone and testosterone.

Signs of hormone imbalance include fatigue, hot flashes, moodiness, weight gain, poor sex drive and poor memory. Most hormonal problems center around estrogen being too high and progesterone too low. This becomes a problem for many women as they get older due to reduced estrogen and progesterone hormones being produced by the endocrine system.

If your estrogen is too high you need to supplement with bioidentical progesterone topical cream to keep progesterone in balance with the higher estrogen.

Too much estrogen can also be the result of a high unfermented soy diet, heredity and obesity or pregnancy.

Self-testing to see if a hormone imbalance exists is available. See HealthCheckUSA.com or 1-800-929-2044.

Hot Flashes (due to menopause)-Take Vitamin B6 and oyster shell calcium, as directed.

Inflammation–Fish oil is helpful against inflamation. It works similarly to ibuprofen. Other items that may be helpful include: fruits, vegetables, curcumin, turmeric, green tea, bromelain (a person who is allergic to either pineapple or pineapple juice should not use bromelain), herb boswella; St John's wort, cat's-claw, white willow, arnica, licorice and niacin. All of the above raise HDL. Also, avoid white sugar and white flour, which react with proteins to create AGES (advance glycation end products). The body compensates for the AGES by producing anti-inflammatory chemicals. Other inflammatory fat includes Omega 6 (grain fed animal meat), baked goods, candy, cereal, margarine, peanut butter and vegetable oil.

Infections—Apply iodine (potassium iodine old style or you can use colloidal silver gel and raw honey by applying both to the wound to prevent it from getting infected. Also, use a sugar and honey mixture; apply it to the infected area, then cover it with gauze. It is necessary to change the dressing everyday.

Another method is to use raw honey or sugar made into a paste with water. Use the gauze with a coating of vaseline around the infected area to create a dam. Then pour the honey or sugar paste into the area and cover with gauze. Change this everyday until the infection disappears. The principle behind this is that bacteria cannot live in a osmotic environment. If the infection is in the intestines, take chamomile tincture(as directed) which helps to prevent constipation and diarrhea.

Insomnia- A person requires the proper amount of sleep to enable the body and the brain to regenerate. Sleep also causes the proteins that accumulate during the day to vanish during the night to permit a person to begin the next day with a clear head.

The herb, Reishi mushrooms is also helpful against insomnia and it also helps to decrease anxiety, along with helping to lower cholesterol. Other herbs that aid in combating insomnia include Valerian root–take as directed before bedtime; skullcap tincture-take as directed. Skullcap can be taken as a tincture or a tea, such as passion flower tea. It is also important to detoxify the liver and the bowels. See the detoxification chapter (Chapter Two)for particulars.

Colloidal Trace Minerals–help to strengthen the nervous system.

Chamomile–available in capsule form and tincture.

Hypothalamus gland support (PMG)–helps to control the body's clock.

Kava Kava–an anti anxiety herb–take as directed, but avoid if pregnancy or depression exists.

Lemon balm-relaxes the body.

Silent Night-a product which is available over the counter. It contains the herbs hops, skullcap and valerian root.

Tryptophan–an amino acid that contains the same ingredient contained in turkey and eggs that makes you seek sleep after a meal. Other supplements that help include Vitamin B complex, particularly Vitamin B-3, melatonin and inositol (take as directed before bedtime.

Joints (Problems with):

Supplements that help include the herb turmeric, which is an antioxidant and anti inflammatory. Other herbs that help include Boswella, ginger and Omega 3 fatty acids. You should also drink herbal tea and green tea for their antioxidants. Also, dehydration can also affect the joints. To avoid dehydration it is recommended that you drink water in proportion to your weight at a rate of your weight times .070. An example: If you weigh 150 pounds, at a minimum you should drink eleven ounces of water each day.

A Magnet wrapped in Velcro, or a copper bracelet, both of which are available over the counter are also helpful in activating the body's electrical signals.

Take DMSO and or MSM for pain and inflammation. MSN is also available with Glucosamine and chondriotin; take as directed. Other helpful supplements include gelatin capsules and sea lipid mussel capsules; take together as directed.

Kidney disease--One source of kidney problems may be the toxic result of metals such as, cadmium, lead, mercury and a variety of environmental pollutants, along with unnatural ingredients that are sometimes added to our food supply.

One particular metal, cadmium, is damaging to the kidneys' tissue. The danger arrives if it is ingested in excessive amounts. Similarly with all metals, weekly detoxification becomes the answer on how to prevent the unwanted accumulation of metals in the body. See also, the Chapter Two on detoxification.

Other suggestions to keep the kidneys healthy: eat red meat moderately and free range when possible. The free range meat will provide better fat (omega 3). Grain-fed meat produces omega 6 fat, which can be inflammatory when eaten in high amounts. Diets that include bad fats may trigger a variety of ailments including high cholesterol and high blood pressure. It is also advisable to avoid high protein diets and processed foods which contain sugar and white flour.

Diets need to contain more complex carbohydrates, vegetables, and fruit to maximize the intake of vitamins minerals and fiber. Fiber is important since it aids indigestion and binds to excess cholesterol, which is taken to excretion. Eating more raw food or slightly cooked food will provide the body with those enzymes that were lost due to over-cooking, yet needed to help fortify the organs and improve the immune system.

Other foods and herbs that work to keep the kidneys healthy include: cranberries; red grapes; grape-seed extract; parsley (a natural diuretic); multi herbal tea and green tea, both of which are antioxidants. Yet other foods and herbs include: Rehmannia root tea; Bupleurum; dandelion (high in potassium) as a tea or leaves included in a salad and the herb horsetail extract.

Yet other supplements, which are helpful, include: high amounts of calcium and magnesium; Vitamin A; Vitamin B complex, particularly Vitamin B 6; amino acid tonic, which contains 21 amino acids that compose the building blocks of metabolism. Several supplements of amino acid liquid are available over the counter.

Kidney Stones–Kidney stones can be caused by too much calcium, poor calcium absorption or a lack of good digestive bacteria (Oxalo), the latter being responsible for breaking down calcium before it reaches the kidneys. Oxalo can be found in sauerkraut, yogurt and other probotics. Also, drinking lemonade helps to dissolve kidney stones. Potassium citrate and magnesium citrate also help to dissolve kidney stones.

A herb called Hydrangea, which is available at many health food stores, dissolves stones. You should also drink cranberry juice often to help make the kidneys alkaline. Dandelion tea is good for detoxification and it helps to maintain phosphorus calcium balance. Magnesium is another supplement that works to dissolve stones and should be taken with a calcium supplement. Zeolite, a natural volcanic substance, is yet another supplement that works to dissolve stones. If not available at your local health food store, it can be obtained online.

Dehydration contributes to a build-up of calcium in the kidneys where stones form. However, keeping hydrated stops the calcium from gathering and reaching a danger-point. If you get a kidney stone, a high-dose potassium supplement will work to dissolve the stone.

Baking soda capsules reduce the build-up of uric acid that can cause the stones to develop. These stones can be the prelude to kidney disease and high blood pressure To ensure the health of the kidneys, the body's blood needs to be alkaline. Another means of reducing the accumulation of calcium is to frequently drink fresh-squeezed lemon juice. It is also helpful to scale-back on proteins and purines which bind with the calcium. By cutting back, less calcium will build-up in the kidneys.

Low calcium diets do not protect against kidney stones. People prone to kidney stones could have excess oxalate production in the stomach which is caused by a low calcium intake. Once the intake of calcium is lowered, the body begins to take calcium from the bones to keep the supply of calcium at its proper level. The depletion of calcium in the bones leads to osteoporosis.

Kidney stones can be caused by an improper diet that includes ingesting too many calcium supplements, combined with a lack of magnesium to keep the calcium liquid in the blood. The stones can also be caused by a lack of sufficient digestive enzymes. Yet another possible cause points to dehydration. If a person becomes dehydrated the undiluted calcium may concentrate and form a stone.

When you keep your body hydrated by drinking plenty of water, the chance of developing kidney stones is greatly lessened. It is also recommended that you cut back on excess calcium intake to prevent oxalate production. And it is recommended that you cut back on salt and animal protein.

Other helpful tips for kidney health include: dandelion tea or dandelion leaves (used in a salad) which aid in detoxification of the kidney; baking soda, mixed with water, should be taken regularly to help reduce the concentration of uric acid in the kidneys. Baking soda also helps to keep the kidneys alkaline, while it also helps to maintain a proper urination flow. In conjunction, a concentration of excess uric acid may lead to kidney stones. It is also helpful to cut back on protein and purines, both of which are found in meats, particularly organ (including heart, liver and intestines). They are also found in mussels, sardines and other seafood.

There are some other options, including the following, which are considered to be old-time remedies that may help:

Option 1–Take seven lemons and squeeze juice of each one separately. Drink the juice of each one during a three-hour period which may dissolve stone.

Option 2- Mix baking soda with water and drink the mixture, which will make the urine less acidic.

Leaky Gut Syndrome--May be due to the bowels being permeated, which leads to proteins (undigested waste) being leaked into the blood stream instead of remaining in the bowel. Food, by remaining in the bowel, keeps the food on tract for proper decomposition and nutrient extraction. However, proteins and waste, by circulating in the blood, can end up in the urine which can cause various complications including fever and inflammation throughout the body. Other complications can lead to asthma, colitis, Crohn's disease, diabetes, lupus, as well as other autoimmune diseases, including rheumatoid arthritis.

The problem with the intestinal tract leakage can be treated by taking probiotics (acidophilus Bifus) in liquid form before meals. Better intestinal bacteria and stomach bacteria can provide proper digestion and a more efficient digestive tract which will work to permit the intestinal lining to heal. Also, in addition to taking the probiotics, you should drink a multi herbal tea, along with taking the supplements, calcium, Colloidal Minerals, magnesium and Vitamin D.

Leukemia–The herb astraglus helps to create immune cells, called macrophages, in bone marrow and in lymph tissue. It is advisable to switch to a completely raw organic diet as often as possible. An all-raw diet increases the amount of enzymes that will be added to your immune system. See also the section on cancer to see the list of herbs that are beneficial in the struggle against Leukemia. Also, add cottage cheese and yogurt to your diet. See also Chapter Two on Detoxification and Listing on PH (page8/9).

Leg pain–Leg pain may be the result of a calcium or potassium deficiency. The herbs kelp and spirulina are helpful in the relief of leg pain. Both serve as a lubricant for the body's joints. Also, gelatin tablets and lipped sea mussels may be helpful in rebuilding cartilage.

Legs, swollen--The herb Job's tears, parsley and watermelon are good diuretics which help to reduce swelling.

Liver Health--Vitamin B12 and Vitamin C, both of which help to fight free radicals and work to keep the liver healthy. Garlic, Panax Ginseng, the herb Tumeric, and Schizandra are blood purifiers and antioxidants that also aid in keeping the liver healthy. Carrots (Vitamin A), Vitamin E (contains antioxidants and lecithin (found naturally in eggs), a supplement that helps metabolize fat. Grapes are good for the kidneys; they fight to prevent the formation of fat.

An over the counter supplement Glucuronate, a nutritional substance, found in leafy green vegetables works to remove toxins from the liver. It binds with toxins (food additives, excess hormones, metals, pesticides, etc;) and carries them to excretion. Another good detoxifier that protects the liver is Milk Thistle; a widely used herb that is known to help with the growth of new liver cells.

Liver health–Suggested supplements include Vitamin E, Milk Thistle Selenium and Lipoic Acid (stimulates the liver cells and helps to curb hepatitis virus). The herb eclipta alba (leaf extract) also helps to stimulate liver cells.

Liver (non-alcoholic fatty liver disease)--is caused by too much fat (triglycerides) and an excessive amount of liver enzymes (free radicals). Taking milk thistle, alpha-lipoic acid and other antioxidants is helpful. It is also helpful to detoxify with bentonite clay, taking Vitamin D and the supplement resveratrol (derivative of red grapes), along with drinking a cup of tea mixed with one drop of liquid lavender daily. Resveratrol helps to accelerate fat metabolism in the liver.

Other supplements that may be helpful: take Alpha Lipoic Acid, an antioxidant that assists in the distribution of other nutrients, such as: Coenzyme Q10, Vitamin C and Vitamin E. Alpha Lipoic Acid also helps to rid the body of arsenic, lead and mercury.

Herbs that are helpful in the fight against liver disease and may help to regenerate liver cells, include the following: Eclipta Alba (also known to afford some protection of the liver from the effects of alcohol) and milk thistle, which acts identically to Eclipta Alba.

Liver detoxification-It is paramount that the liver gets detoxified of fats and toxins that accumulate. Detoxification transports the fats and toxins to the gallbladder which breaks the matter down by adding salt and enzymes before passing it along to the intestines for excretion. The following options may help:

→**Oregon grape extract**–Use as a tea–It requires about 12 weeks to work. The extract is also available in topical form for psoriasis.

→**Calendula herb with olive oil**--mix together and combine it with red clover, chick weed and horsetail tinctures--drink it, mixed with tea.

→**Multi herbal tea with 1 drop of organic lavender**–take daily for two weeks and afterward, take twice a week for maintenance.

→**Cod Liver Oil**-use cod liver oil to cleanse your digestive tract.

→**Beet juice**, burdock root or Rhubarb root and dandelion are also helpful.

Lupus--fresh pineapple contains bromelain a natural anti-inflammatory or take the supplement bromelain, combined with a strict vegetarian diet. It is important that with the diet, you must avoid eating meat, which can make your blood acidic. Dairy products, including eggs, create arachidonic acid (Omega 6), which in turn creates inflammation. Also wheat (gluten) triggers the blood to create antibodies, which can attack good cells and cause an auto-immune problem. You should eat fish frequently and take Vitamin E (as directed on label). Vitamin C also helps to keep the effects of Lupus less severe. Also, some foods, including fruits and vegetable may still contain insecticide (spray) and the best way to protect yourself is to eat organic fruits and vegetables. Foods that contain any type of insecticide may trigger lupus. (See also Chapter Two on Detoxification and listing for PH on page 8/9).

Lymph system--Cleansing the lymph system–The lymph is a system of fluid filled pockets (nodes) that includes bone marrow, blood vessels, ducts, glands, spleen, liver and tonsils. Each of them act as a purifying collection station for old red blood cells and toxins, which are then excreted from the body.

The lymph system gets bogged down when it has to process unnatural (man-made) foods. It is important to keep the lymph system flowing and this can be accomplished by drinking plenty of water, eating raw vegetables and fruit and drinking non-sugared fruit juice. Other things that help to support the lymph system include the following supplements: essential fatty acids (fish oil and flax seed). A multi-herbal tea that contains echinacea is another beneficial supplement. It is also important that you exercise regularly, primarily because the lymph system is put into motion, solely by body movement.

Lymph System (Lymph Flush)--Calendula herb infused with olive oil should be combined with dandelion root, red clover, chick weed, and horsetail. Take the combination as a tea on a daily basis for one week.

The immune system can operate at maximum efficiency through the foods we eat. Using herbs is an excellent way to provide the body with necessary nutrients including antioxidants, enzymes, minerals and vitamins all of which fight against invading intruders. Herbs are alkalizing to the body and they function to keep our PH alkaline, which helps to prevent an unnatural acidic environment. If your body is alkaline you essentially have a shield (oxygen rich body tissue and blood) which works to resist bacteria and viruses.

Once the body is alkaline, it has prepared itself with what can be described as an unfriendly environment for any invading intruders. One of the best methods of making the body alkaline is by eating vegetables, preferably raw and hefty portions of fruit. Another item that is beneficial in the process is to drink apple cider vinegar or take an apple cider vinegar supplement. Also, you do not need to totally exclude red meat; however, it should be eaten in moderation to prevent the blood from becoming acidic.

Macular Degeneration--Macular Degeneration effects a small portion of the eye, the macula, which controls color and the optic nerve signals that are necessary for vision, particularly sharp detail. At present, there is no cure for the disease, which is thought to be caused by a failure of the immune system.

When faced with the disease, although no cure is yet available, there are measures that can be taken to forestall the pace of the disease. Taking offensive action is preferable to taking no action, which would automatically place you on the defensive as the disease progresses. The following suggestions may be helpful:

Eat plenty of fruit for antioxidants; eat eggs for lutein (helps to clear the blood vessels); eat hefty portions of leafy green vegetables; however, carrots are also extremely beneficial for the eyes. In the event you prefer not to eat carrots, take the supplement beta carotene (as directed on label). Trace minerals or Colloidal Minerals and a high power multivitamin, particularly one that contains a high dosage of Vitamin A.

Other supplements and herbs that are helpful in dealing with macular degeneration include the following: taurine; bilberry (helps to improve circulation to the eyes), Vitamin C, Vitamin D, gingko biloba, lipoic acid and Co Q10. It is also important to eliminate sugar, vegetable oil, white flour products and processed foods from your diet. Yet other helpful things to do include wearing sunglasses when you are out in the sun to block the glare. Also, with regard to taking the herb bilberry, you can make tea from the herb and drink several cups a day.

Yet other supplements that can be taken include: fish oil (contains Omega 3 and it helps to reduce the risk of macular degeneration); nuts (almonds, pecans and walnuts also contain Omega 3 and vitamins); cantaloupe (contains high amounts of beta-carotene, which converts to Vitamin A, which is very good for the eyes); Bell peppers (high in Vitamin C).

Also, with regard to the earlier mentioned leafy green vegetables it should be noted that spinach and leafy green vegetables are rich in Lutein, which helps the pigment in the macular section of the eye. They also helps to fight cell oxidation which has been noted as a leading cause of macular degeneration. In addition, the leafy greens also work to protect the eyes from the glare of the sun's rays.

Memory–DMAE (Deanol), which is found in sardines, increases production of choline in the brain and it also increases the production of acetylcholine (neurotransmitter in both the peripheral nervous system and central nervous system), which improves memory and reduces hyperactivity.

➔**Lecithin capsules**–may improve memory.

➔**Acetyl-L-carnitine**–is an amino acid that may help in reversing the aging process in brain cells. It is also good for the heart and the muscles.

➔ **Gingko Biloba**–May increase memory by dilating blood vessels.

➔**Coenzyme Q10**, which is helpful to circulation; L-carnitine; flavonoids, fish oil (omega 3). Red Grapes, red wine and cocoanut oil are also good for circulation. Cocoanut oil is capable of crossing the blood-brain barrier (MCT–medium chain triglyceride) to provide energy to brain cells.

➔Stay away from sugar substitutes, which are known to reduce oxygen in the blood, particularly in the brain. The sugar substitutes may also cause the insulin to be secreted which can trick the pancreas into producing insulin because it is falsely expecting sugar (glucose). When the pancreas fails to receive the sugar it expected, the blood, which is full of insulin, has no where to go. Consequently, lactic acid begins to build up in the brain, which in turn causes the neurons in the brain to begin to die. Also, sugar substitutes, which are unnatural products can also be the cause of headaches, including migraines.

Menopause–Add four tablespoons of ground flaxseed on cereal or yogurt, which will help with hot flashes. If you are experiencing hot flashes, it may be a sign of high cholesterol. Also, if you suffer from cramps, the herb cramp bark tincture may be helpful. Take as directed (on days when the cramps are severe).

Menstruation–Chaste treeberry extract tincture is helpful for the relief of PMS. It helps to normalize menstrual cycles, particularly in young women. Other helpful herbs for menstrual cramps are: cramp bark, ginger and motherwort.

Mouth Ulcer--Drinking calendula tea which is antibacterial and antiviral.

Muscles (sore)–Use Braggs' amino acid mix which will help to relieve sore muscles. The mix will also help to regenerate muscles after exercising (work out, etc.). Also, vinegar helps to remove lactic acid that builds up after exercising or a period of hard work.

Multiple Sclerosis (MS)-MS is considered to be an autoimmune disease that causes self destruction of the protective nerve coating called myelin. The loss of the myelin sheathing exposes the nerves to damage. This self destruction is thought to be similar to Rheumatoid arthritis where killer cells attack good cells thinking they are pathogens.

People in colder climates are more susceptible to MS as opposed to warmer climates where the disease is rare. It is possible that the warmer temperatures cause the disease to occur less often and support the theory that a Vitamin D deficiency could be a trigger.

It is important that you expose your body (face and hands) to the sun on a daily basis to allow the body to absorb Vitamin D. If you are unable to get out in the sunlight, you can purchase Vitamin D3 as a supplement.

Triggers can also be caused by toxic accumulations in the body and poor digestion that impedes nutrient assimilation. Other triggers can be food allergies caused by processed foods and the additives associated with this type of food. Your diet should include an increase in the amount of fish you consume. Your diet should also include fiber, fruit (for antioxidants), raw vegetables and organic foods. It is also important to eliminate fried food, white flour, white sugar and limit your consumption of meat.

Supplements should include; fish oil, flax seed oil, cod liver oil, and borage oil should be taken to provide fatty acids. The fatty acids help create the myelin sheathing which protects the nerves. Other helpful supplements include a product known as Super Green Food (for nutritional support), Vitamin B-complex and Vitamin B-12, which supports the immune system.

Other supplements include a high quality multi-herbal tea, which contains nutrients; Ginkgo Biloba, which supports the blood vessels; Colloidal Minerals, which contains the 74 minerals that are usually deficient in many people; high potency multi-vitamins and the Herb ashwagandha (contains ingredients that aid against stress and helps balance hormones).

Also, digestive enzymes like yogurt, sauerkraut, and acidophilus work to improve digestion and nutrient assimilation.

Equally importantly, it is necessary to keep the body detoxified by ridding the body of toxic material. This can be accomplished with one drop of lavender included in a cup of herbal tea. Drink the tea on a daily basis for two weeks and afterward, drink one cup of the tea every third day to help keep the liver detoxified. To help eliminate toxic chemicals from the body, use bentonite clay (one teaspoon mixed with water; drink every three days). Some foods that help to detoxify the body are radishes and dandelion root. Also, over the counter cleansers are available. See detoxification chapter (Chapter Two).

Night sweats and hot flashes– Take bee pollen wafers and evening primrose oil in the evening.

Nose bleeds- could be bioflavonoid deficiency–Good sources of bio flavonoids, which strengthen the capillaries of the body, are dark fruits, including blackberries, blueberries and plums.

Osteoarthritis – otherwise known as joint pain caused by cartilage loss can be the result of too much calcium intake. This forms excess calcium deposits which can be eliminated by taking a magnesium supplement including Vitamin D and the minerals Boron, Copper and Strontium. In the event of cartilage loss, gelatin (Jello), and the supplements sea lipped muscles and silica are helpful. Other helpful over the counter products include Arnica cream or tablets, oregano oil or the dried herb oregano, gamma linolenic acid capsules (a fatty acid) and fish oil (omega 3).

Osteoporosis - A lack of calcium to the body will cause the body to pull its calcium needs from the bones. Strong bones need food rich in calcium like leafy green vegetables (broccoli, romaine lettuce), nuts (have isoflavonoids to allow more calcium absorption), seeds, and fish. Soda, caffeine, salt and alcohol contribute to the bone breakdown if taken in excess. The need for weight bearing exercise can halt bone loss because it stimulates bone cell formation. Also, osteoporosis is an acid problem. The more acidic you are the more the body's defense uses calcium to get you alkaline. Stay away from salt and carbonated soda, both of which deplete calcium.

Suggested supplements:

Boron–helps to metabolize Vitamin D and it reduces the excretion of calcium. If you lack sufficient calcium, it may be due to a diet which contains too much protein. The excess protein creates acid by-products that extract calcium from the bones to maintain the body's alkalinity. Coral calcium (available with the ingredients required for absorption).

Magnesium is required for calcium absorption. Magnesium also activates enzymes which aid in normal bone development.

The following supplements are also helpful: Vitamin D; Vitamin K (needed to attract calcium to the bone marrow); Fish Oil (improves calcium absorption); Silica (hardens the bones and it is also beneficial for the teeth and the gums); Strontium–a trace mineral that acts as concrete for the bones.

If you suffer from osteoporosis, the following diet, rich in calcium may help. Eat foods like dandelion, bok choy, orange juice, apple juice, cabbage, sardines, and broccoli. Western diets contain too much protein and dairy. This causes the blood to be acidic (acidosis) causing the bodies biological system to deplete magnesium and calcium from the bones in order to balance the natural alkalinity with the ever present acidity. This calcium loss occurs through urination. Also, sugar extracts calcium and vitamins from the bones and disrupts the calcium phosphorous balance.

PMS (Premenstrual Syndrome) – Take the amino acid Phenlalanine before your period starts. It is good for cramps, mood swings and body aches. Magnesium is necessary for the metabolism of estrogen and relieves cramping (take as directed). Vitamin B6 works with magnesium for estrogen metabolism in the liver. Calcium helps prevent PMS.

If you have severe PMS add natural progesterone to your regimen. Apply natural progesterone cream to the inside of the forearm and wrist beginning after ovulation until one day before your period starts. Stay away from sugar as it depletes the minerals in your body. Stop eating sugar two weeks before your period starts. If you retain water, cut back on salt. Eat lots of fiber. Stay away from animal products with hormones and keep your diet low in fats during this period, because saturated fat increases estrogen levels.

PMS Pain: The following are helpful when dealing with PMS pain: borage oil, which contains linoleic acid, is anti-inflammatory and fish oil is also an anti-inflammatory. Other helpful supplement are MSM, Korean angelica and elderberry tea or tincture.

Pancreatic Cancer –See Cancer Pancreatic (Page 92).

Parkinson's Disease--a degeneration of the nerves in the brain. The cause of the disease is unknown; however. the end results are low dopamine (L dopa) levels and an imbalance of Acetylcholine. The disease itself has increased immensely since 1970. Its cause seems to be related to either a dietary or environmental toxin. It has also been suspected that drug pesticides, heavy metals and other pollutants raise the body's toxicity and cause free radicals to find a home in tissue from where the radicals initiate their destructive process.

There are drugs to deal with this disease but there are side effects associated with them. Nonetheless, under any circumstances, you will want to strengthen your body. The following suggestions will be instrumental in achieving that goal.

➔ Detoxification to rid body of toxins (see Chapter Two on detox).

➔ Good diet of fruits and vegetables plus plenty of fiber to aid in detoxification.

➔ Good digestion-take the following; supplement digestive enzymes, yogurt, sauerkraut or liquid acidophilus. Good digestion improves good nutrient absorption and bowel movements (detox). Eat as much raw food as possible to acquire enzymes that are normally lost in cooking. Also, eat lots of beans and wild fish (not farmed) for protein and Omega 3 oils. Avoid fast food (junk food), sugar, white flour and processed foods.

Supplements include:

→A Good multi vitamin; Colloidal Minerals or trace minerals.

→A bean that contains L Dopa is the velvet bean. Evening primrose contains tryptophan, an amino acid, that aids L-Dopa to turn into dopamine. Take as directed.

→Ginkgo Biloba--good for circulation.

→Passion flower–contains alkaloids and nicotine. It increases the production of dopamine.

The disease essentially causes a deterioration of the nerves that control movement in the brain. It is thought that those who suffer from Parkinson's disease are also deficient in Vitamins B 2, B 6 and B12.

An old time remedy that may be helpful--boil the following in 4 quarts of water for 2 minutes and drink often; Peach tree leaves 2 cups; Passion flower 1 cup; Bugle weed 1 cup; Catnip1 cup and Mullein 1 cup.

People who smoke rarely come down with Parkinson's disease because the tobacco depletes the buildup of monoamine oxidase, which regulates neurotransmitters. Too much monoxide is associated with Parkinson's and those who smoke are less susceptible to Parkinson's Disease.

Pituitary gland support- Pituitrophin pmg, a bovine extract, which supports the pituitary gland and is responsible for body growth and various hormonal functions. Take as directed. Fish oil and chiro seed also support the pituitary gland.

Polmonary embolism-A clot blocks an artery in the lungs. It initially occurs when the area around the mouth turns blue. Simultaneously, you will have some trouble breathing.

Poison Ivy – Use bleach, mixed with water. Apply to the affected area to dry out the poison ivy.

Prostate (Health of)–It is important to maintain a healthy prostate and the primary step required is that the body must be detoxified to eliminate toxins from causing harm (See Chapter Two on Detoxification). Secondly, it is equally important that the body be alkaline (See Chapter One). Diet is also extremely important, particularly consumption of sugar, which should be kept at a minimum. Another helpful item is baking soda. Mix 1/4 teaspoon with a glass of water and take once a day, which will help to keep the prostate and the bladder alkaline. It is equally important that you design a diet that includes high amounts of raw fruits, vegetables and fiber.

Your diet should also include multi grain bread, rather than white bread; beans; cottage cheese; garlic; grains, wheat pasta, wild rice, sauerkraut and yogurt. Raw foods contain high amounts of enzymes and good digestive bacteria. Grapes, red and black, contain high amounts of antioxidants. Other dietary considerations should include herbal tea and essential minerals, such as Colloidal Minerals and trace minerals which contain all the necessary minerals needed to maintain a good immune system.

Sugar, when consumed in excess amounts, is not absorbed properly in the body. Rather, it winds up in the liver where it is transformed into triglycerides which are implicated in the development of cancer. Refined sugar naturally triggers insulin and when it is constantly created, every organ is affected by the inflammatory side effects.

Olestra, the artificial fat used by some manufacturers in such foods as potato chips is thought to be responsible for lowering blood levels of some carotenoids, including licopenes, which are vital in the fight against prostate cancer. Another caution is that excessive consumption of alcoholic beverages can also be detrimental in the struggle against prostate cancer. Moderation, when drinking, should be the rule. Excessive drinking can also cause severe side effects in general and they are not limited to the prostate.

The diet should include foods that are high in fiber. The fiber helps to reduce cholesterol levels and also reduces testosterone levels.

Other foods that bolster the prostate include blueberries, red grapes (with seeds), raw garlic and multi-herbal tea. Supplements that help the prostate include: Colloidal Minerals (contains selenium, a protector of the prostate), zinc, Vitamin D, Vitamin E; fish oil; sal palmetto and a good multi-vitamin.

Herbs that are known to be helpful remedies include: nettle root extract, which can also be taken as a cocktail (herb combination or cocktail sal palmetto, echineacia nettle root, cramp bark and chamomile); rye pollen extract.

Other helpful remedies include: winter huckleberry tea; New Jersey tea root (also called redshank); fish oil; lycopene; juniper berries (helpful for swollen prostate) and corn silk tea a detoxifying diuretic. Walnuts are also a helpful food. They are rich in Omega 3 and other nutrients that aid in prostate health. Stinging Nettle extract is also helpful because it raises the levels of free testosterone.

Prostate (cancer)--Cancer patients should maintain a daily diet that is confined to healthy foods that include: fruits, vegetables, breads, oatmeal, grain products, brown or wild rice, pasta or beans (rich in fiber) several times a day, lean poultry. It is recommended that the day's consumption of liquid should include cranberry juice (not cranberry drink or cocktail, both of which contain high amounts of sugar) and plenty of water, along with sugar-free juice.

Some helpful foods: Broccoli and cauliflower are each beneficial to cancer survivors. The soluble fiber contained in vegetables works to lower levels of testosterone, while it slows the progression of prostate cancer. Beans, which are rich in fiber, are extremely effective. Garlic which contains anti-cancer properties is also helpful.

Deep water fish should be eaten to avoid toxins associated with surface fish and bottom scavengers. It is also necessary to remember that fish oil, although healthy for the body, when taken in large doses could possibly suppress the immune system.

Grapes (and grape seed extract)--grapes are recognized as an antioxidant food and darker (red) grapes are known to be the best choice in strengthening the immune system. Green tea is also helpful. It contains polyphenols, which support scavenger cells in ridding the body of free radicals.

Miatake mushrooms are beneficial. They form a strong immune stimulant which works to inhibit the growth of tumors. The mushrooms are available in capsules. Fermented soy protein is known as a formidable enemy of prostate cancer. Japanese men, who consume the protein have a lower rate of death due to prostate cancer. Pumpkin seeds, a healthy food which is rich in zinc and contain magnesium and oleic acid which may help urine to more easily flow.

Strawberries and blueberries contain strong antioxidant properties. Blueberries are also known to combat night-blindness.

Tomatoes are a source of lycopene, an anti-oxidant. Lycopene is a carotenoid and may be the most potent antioxidant for the fight against prostate cancer. Lycopene may reduce the risk of prostate cancer by almost 45 percent. Apparently the most effective source for the substance is tomato-based products that have been cooked with a small amount of oil(preferably olive oil). Tomato sauce and pizza are much more effective than plain tomatoes or tomato juice. Also, placing a little olive oil in the cooking process seems to enhance the absorption of lycopene.

Other antioxidants that are helpful include: Beta Carotene; grape seed extract; Vitamin C; Vitamin E; pycnogenol and Selenium. Beta Carotene is the best supplement to take because of its ability to convert itself into Vitamin A. Beta Carotene also helps the body to protect itself from free radicals by acting as a fighter against cancer.

Other supplements that are beneficial for prostate health include: CoQ10 (sometimes called Vitamin Q), which is a powerful antioxidant; sal palmetto; Vitamin C; Vitamin D (research has shown that men with lower levels of Vitamin D are more prone to developing prostate cancer) and Vitamin E. It is known that semen, when left dormant can cause difficulties because it can deteriorate and create cell-mutation.

Saturated fats such as butter; bacon; range fed red meat, are not an issue. Some studies have shown that people, including Eskimos, who live the longest and healthiest maintain diets that are high in saturated fat. Those same people usually have cholesterol levels of around 350. Also, brown seaweed, which contains Fucoxanthin, has shown to be effective in helping to reduce cancer cells.

Consumption of refined white sugar or foods high in sugar by people suffering from cancer are essentially eating foods that actually produce food for the pernicious cancer cells.

Benign Prostatic Hyperplasia (swollen prostate)–Supplements that may be helpful include: multi herbal tea; sal palmetto; pygeum africanum; fish oil; flaxseed oil; zinc; beta carotine (Vitamin A); Vitamin C; beta sitosterol; selenium (trace minerals); stinging nettle root; rye pollen extract; licorice tincture (helps to prevent the conversion of testosterone to dihydrotestosterone); pumpkin seeds (helps the flow of urine).

It is also important to drink plenty of water to flush the kidneys and detoxify toxins produced by processed foods; refrain from sugar which helps to cause prostate disorders to become more serious. Caffeine is known to cause the same effects as sugar. However, Organic cranberry juice (sugarless), an over-the-counter product, is known to be helpful.

Ezee flow tea, is helpful and yet another supplement, glycine, is an amino acid which helps to reduce an enlarged prostate and works to help detoxify the liver.

The keys to maintaining proper control of the prostate must include detoxification and the following: proper hormone balance through diet; exercise and nutritional supplements. Detoxification is very important because some toxins disrupt the estrogen testosterone balance in men. Adding a high fiber diet also helps to detoxify the body, while it also helps eliminate excess cholesterol.

Psoriasis – Cells replicate ten times faster than normal. The causes are unknown, but could be genetic flaws or poor diets. For relief, add a couple of capfuls of vegetable oil to your bath water towards the end of your bath. It will keep the water from drying out your skin. Also, before entering the bathtub, add magnesium to the water. The magnesium is an electrolyte that is very good for the health of the skin's cells.

Many people travel to the Dead Sea, known to contain magnesium, to soak themselves to help eliminate various skin related problems. Also, take olive oil, for 2 months and use either Vitamin D or Vitamin D cream, curcumin (herb) and fish oil. Curry and zinc are also helpful.

Psoriasis can also be caused by food allergies and poor liver function. Use lavender, tea tree oil or a calendula salve for the liver. Other supplements include milk thistle; burdock root and Omega 3 (fish oil). In conjunction, people in Germany often use Witch Hazel, aloe vera, tea tree oil, oil of clove and cedar leaf oil as a remedy. Once the psoriasis subsides, drink gotu kola tea to help heal the tissue under the skin. Another useful option is to use Oregon grape seed extract topically.

Psoriasis can also be caused by a thyroid condition, since the thyroid controls skin cell replacement. It is advisable to avoid red meat. Both red meat and milk contain arachidonic acid, which aggravates inflammation. People who suffer from Psoriasis usually have poor or incomplete digestion, which can cause the creation of toxins known as polyamines. These polyamines can lead to the proliferation of skin cells and cause the over growth of Candidacies (yeast infection) which might also cause psoriasis. Garlic and oregano oil both work effectively to eliminate yeast infection.

Also, there is a relationship between psoriasis and lack of fatty acids, thus the need for fish oil and flax oil. Also, adding sea salt to the bath water is beneficial and works to heal the skin. A substitute for sea salt is vinegar, which can be added to the bath water or be applied directly to the skin.

Psoriasis also makes it necessary to detoxify the body, especially the liver, since it filters toxins from the body. One helpful way is to fast for three days on a diet of juice supplemented by drinking large amounts of water, green tea and herbal teas. Other supplements to be added to the diet include fish oil and hydrochloric acid tablets, both of which should be taken before each meal to aid in digestion.

Other supplements include: Vitamin A, Vitamin B complex, Colloidal Minerals, milk thistle, multivitamins and zinc. Acidophilus and generous amounts of leafy green vegetables should be added to the diet. They (green leafy vegetables) contain chlorophyll which is extremely beneficial to the skin. Also, selenium (colloidal mineral) keeps the skin smooth and prevents dandruff.

Some over the counter products that combat psoriasis include Zostrix, which supplements treatment for shingles (a form of psoriasis); use as directed to help eliminate inflammation. Another product is Cholacol, which works to supply bile salt and helps to remove intestinal toxins. Usually, people suffering from psoriasis have a deficiency in bile salt. Psoriasis can also emerge as a side effect due to synthetic hormone replacement in menopausal women. The condition (synthetic hormone replacement) may also cause skin irritation.

Rash – allergic reaction to food, stress, or makeup. Clear skin with witch hazel and apply aloe vera. Toxins can also cause a rash, making it important to detox the liver of metals and toxins with one teaspoon of bentonite clay, mixed with water. Also, give yourself a lymph massage to get the lymph moving faster to clear out toxins. Exercise also keeps the lymph system in motion. In addition, using a hair brush on the skin activates the skin cells to detoxify the body.

Restless Leg Syndrome –May be caused by a toxic buildup in the leg muscles, which results from an overloaded liver. It is then necessary to detox the liver. Supplements that may help include reduced glutathione and milk thistle.

Rheumatoid Arthritis – has been linked to a deficiency of the amino acid tyrosine, which helps to metabolize proteins. The body manufactures tyrosine and it is also obtained from foods including: beans, cheese, cottage cheese, chicken, nuts, turkey and yogurt. It is also a fat burner and mood enhancer that transmits signals between cells, which can help those who suffer from RA.

Ring Worm–There are two over-the-counter products available that are effective against Ring Worm, Butemafine or Terbinafine. Also, the herb Golden Seal Root (powder form) is effective; mix with water to make a paste and apply as needed.

Rosacea–Usually noticeable in middle aged people, especially women. Something triggers the rush of blood to the facial area which is the result of blood vessel dilation. In people with rosacea, the blood vessels do not constrict causing the blood vessels to stay dilated. What the triggers are is the key to solving the problem. The following are possible triggers: Alcohol; Food Allergies; Poor digestion (most common); Nutrient deficiencies (also common); Hormone imbalance.

Skin problems are usually one of the body's signals that something is wrong internally. The most common problem is due to poor digestion, usually associated with acid reflux as a side effect. This is a lack of stomach acid (hydrochloric acid) necessary for food digestion and a lack of good digestive system bacteria, which aids in digestion and nutrient assimilation. Also, detox the skin with Witch Hazel and apply aloe vera after detoxification.

The following supplements may help: take (HCL) hydrochloric acid tablets as directed; eat 1 tablespoon of raw unheated sauerkraut before each meal for good bacteria; use grape seed extract cream on the area as an anti-inflammatory. Also, horse chestnut cream can be used to shrink veins.

Eat yogurt often to acquire good bacteria. Liquid acidophilus is also an excellent source of good bacteria. Take before meals as directed.

Detoxify body –Toxins that are stored in the body's fat and body tissue try to exit the skin. Poor digestion requires detoxification. See Also Chapter Two on detoxification.

Drink a multi-herbal tea for nutrients and detoxification.

Other helpful supplements include:

→A good multivitamin.

→Vitamin B-complex.

→Take Vitamin B-12 sublingually – 2 times daily.

→Milk thistle capsules – an herb that protects the liver and aids in detoxification.

→Drink lots of water to help with detoxification.

→Eat plenty of fiber to help with detoxification and to help carry off excess cholesterol and toxins.

→Burdock root – a good detoxification herb.

→Hormone imbalance--Low progesterone or birth control pills may be the cause of the skin problem. If you use hormone replacement therapy make sure it is all natural.

Scalp Fungus – three raw cloves of garlic or garlic capsules daily for 9 weeks if necessary. Goldenseal (also available for topical application) and the herb Oregon grape root (taken internally) are recommended; take as directed. Another available product is Chaparral leaf (salve). If you are using a salve, it is recommended that you also use an internal herb such as Echinacea to help fight the fungus from the inside.

Shingles – (herpes virus) Take olive leaf capsules and oregano oil P-73. It is also helpful to include apple cider vinegar, Vitamin C, B12 (sublingual type), zinc, a multi-vitamin and Vitamin A. An over the counter product, Zostrix, fights the substance chemical (Zoster virus) that initiates shingles. Use it for three weeks (according to directions on the label) to eliminate the skin plaque and inflammation. You can take a product called Olivus, which is anti-viral. Take as directed. If you never had Chicken Pox as a child, shingles is contagious.

Skin--Vitamin D is naturally acquired from the sun's rays. It is necessary to get out in the sunshine for about 20-30 minutes every day, which will produce thousands of IU of Vitamin D. The supplement, Vitamin D should be a vital part of your diet, particularly if you are unable to get out in the sun (all seasons). It is through the skin's epidermis that the latent Vitamin D, through a chemical reaction, becomes Vitamin D 3, which aids in defending against foreign invaders (pathogens).

Vitamin D supplements are fat soluble, which prevent the supplements from being absorbed unless they are taken along with some form of fat, including meat, milk or olive oil. Also, the fact that the skin has the ability to recover from oxidation, is due to the fatty acids that are contained in the body. In conjunction, the body's cells reproduce by about 30,000 every minute.

Topical Vitamin D can also be used on skin injuries and for Vitamin D absorption. Topical creams that have alpha lipoic acid are anti-aging which protects against free radicals and a great antioxidant. Also, Vitamin D and Vitamin D 3 lotions help to offset the loss of thousands of cells per minute.

Liquid grape seed extract and Vitamin C are good anti-oxidants and skin healers for eczema and psoriasis. Vitamin E protects from UV damage against free radicals and oxidation of fats in the cell membranes.

A lack of silica which is stored in the hair and skin leads to thinning hair. A deficiency in silica can also cause acne, psoriasis and poor bone strength. Use the herb calendula (in tincture), which contains carotenoids, for rashes and wounds. It also protects the liver and kidneys.

Skin Anti-aging – Plants can provide protection to the skin from aging, skin cancer and sunburn. A plant extract from a fern, Polypodium Leucotomos, is an antioxidant, which enhances the skins collagen. It is used by natives of Honduras to protect against sun and UV damage, Psoriasis and other skin inflammations. This product has a lot of polyphenols, which help the skin retain its moisture and elasticity. The herb ashwagandha also combats aging by reducing cortisol levels, which are known to increase during times of great stress.

Skin (Dry) –Dry skin is usually due to a lack of essential fatty acids. Refrain from eating acidic foods. Take Colloidal Minerals, a high potency multi vitamin and flax seed. Also, take digestive enzymes for nutrient absorption. Use topical cream for dry skin, liquid vitamin C and grape seed extract mixed together. Also, Detox is important. Take Omega 3, selenium, Vitamins A, B complex, D, E , A and zinc.

Skin infection–use a petroleum jelly with a pinch of tree resin. If unavailable from a store, it can be obtained online at www.natrhealth.com. Another remedy that can be used is honey or sugar mixed with honey. Pour the honey into a strip of gauze, coated with vaseline, to keep the honey in place. Afterward, wrap the infected area with the gauze.

Skin problem – Skin problems usually indicate an internal problem. Detoxification is necessary to remove toxins from the body. It is equally helpful to eat lemons, which helps the detoxification. Lemons also contain high amounts of Vitamin C. It is also helpful to wash the skin with vinegar.

You can also combine the lemons and vinegar, mixed with a cup of herbal tea and drink one cup per day. Adding one drop of lavender in the tea for two weeks aid the liver detoxification. After the first two weeks, add one drop of lavender to the tea every 3rd day for maintenance. Also, you can detox with the supplements Reduced Glutathione and milk thistle. Bentonite clay, mixed with a little water, also kills bacteria and pathogens, which can develop resistance to antibiotics, but not against clay. You can also use Yucca powder to bind harmful fats and toxins and pass them to excretion.

Sinus Infection–-adding peppermint oil to a vaporizer may help clear the sinuses. Also, wild cherry bark tea is good for the sinuses. Another item, P-73 oregano oil, which is available in liquid form to be taken by mouth. However, oregano oil is also available in a spray product called Orega Spray (to be taken by spraying into the nostrils). Salt water can also be taken up the nostrils, one at time, by tilting your head and pouring into your nostril. It is important to remember to keep your chin tilted upwards to prevent the salt water from running down your throat. Repeat the process two or three times to help clear the sinuses by breaking up the mucus. The salt water also helps to clear up an infection.

Sleep problem–Take magnesium and calcium (as directed), which helps the body make serotonin. The serotonin makes melatonin, which helps your internal clock and releases transmitters to initiate relaxation.

Smokers–Support your immune system if you smoke. Some examples include taking folic acid, which protects the blood vessels and improves the elasticity of arteries. CoQ10, an antioxidant, that helps to protect heart. Also, people who drink red wine are known to have a lower risk of getting lung cancer.

Reduce the chance of having a stroke by cleaning the blood vessels of plaque and strengthening the arteries. Plaque reduction can be helped through antioxidants such as celery and garlic. Also, trace minerals or colloidal minerals, along with ginkgo biloba helps to dilate the blood vessels to accommodate more circulation of blood.

Sore gums–If due to wearing dentures use Vitamin E complex two times per day.

Stress-The following herbs may be used to decrease stress: cayenne, ginger, gotu kola, sage, turmeric, mixed together and used on food for seasoning or mix with water. Another herb that is useful in combating stress is Panax ginseng. In conjunction, Germany's equivalent to the U.S. FDA commission approves using Panax ginseng to relieve fatigue. Panax ginseng is also available in capsule form; take as directed. It is recommended in Germany to continue using for three consecutive weeks, followed by not taking it for one week. Afterward, if you repeat the process, always take for three weeks followed by a one week break. Also, do not take if you are diabetic or if you are on blood thinners, have high blood pressure, or if you are pregnant.

Schisandra is an herb (Chinese berry) that has been used for centuries by monks to help reduce stress. It is not quite as strong as Panax Ginseng, however, it is softer and tastier. Schisandra is also an antioxidant, which may help to improve a person's mental performance, while it works to protect the liver.

The herb milk thistle works to coat and protect the liver. Its use is suggested for anyone who is under stress or any of the following: drinking alcohol, using pharmaceutical drugs, exposure to pesticides, automobile toxins, and fumes from other sources. Milk Thistle is also a free radical scavenger that helps maintain glutathione levels.

Stress puts strain on the adrenal glands if the condition continues over a long period of time, the glands will be unable to function properly. Consuming too much refined sugar or natural sugar, which is contained in raw fruit, can bring about the same effect. Processed foods can also strain the adrenal glands and deplete the body of Vitamin B 6, which helps detox metals. Constant stress also leads to poor digestion and poor nutrition. You can relieve the problem by taking probotics (digestive enzymes like liquid acidophilus) and by reducing your sugar intake. Also, Vitamin C, the herb gotu kola and ginkgo biloba are good for the adrenal glands. It is also recommended that you drink lemon water frequently to help keep your kidneys functioning properly.

Adrenal gland stress can be helped with a product called Drenamin. Take as directed before each meal on an empty stomach, plus take a high potency multi-vitamin, B complex and B12 taken separately. Note: B6 deficiency is linked to less neurotransmitter production, which is essentially a lack of dopamine, which helps relieve stress.

Tea of skull cap, chamomile, kava kava and passionflower can be used as a combination (tea) to support the adrenal glands.

Stroke and Clot Reducers – include the following: Ginkgo biloba 80mg -4 times daily; garlic - three raw cloves daily; Hawthorne, 250mg daily. The herbs ginger and alfalfa are also helpful and should be taken daily.

Sugar Cravings–usually caused by a deficiency of chromium. A good supplemental source of chromium is contained in Colloidal Minerals. However, an alternate source of chromium can be purchased in liquid or tablet form. Take as directed on label.

Sunburn – Add baking soda and oatmeal to the bath water. Another helpful way to ease the pain of sunburn is to apply hot tea from a wash cloth (team compresses) over the burns. Also, some other remedies that help against sunburn are Aloe Vera gel; mix white vinegar and apple cider vinegar in a container and spray directly on the sunburn. Other sources that may be used include capsules of gotu kola which helps to stimulate skin cells to regenerate and to repair the skin. Liquid Vitamin C, mixed with Vitamin E and applied topically is also helpful.

For a natural sunscreen, eat more carotenoids (kale, carrots, sweet potatoes), lycopenes (tomatoes) and Omega 3. Also, use a sunscreen made with zinc oxide and titanium oxide. The other sunscreens are full of chemicals and get absorbed into blood and may disrupt hormone activity.

Swollen Ankles–See Ankles, swollen.

Swollen Legs –See Legs, swollen.

Teeth Plaque–Brushing with baking soda and hydrogen peroxide kills germs and plaque. Also, fresh strawberries clean teeth of plaque. Also, chewing raw garlic kills germs and you should also eat apples which are natural teeth cleaners.

Tendonitis -Refrain from trans fats (fried foods); they interfere with the fatty acid that helps promote healthy joints. The following herbs are helpful: boswella, cayenne curcumin, magnesium and turmeric.

Thyroid–Basal Rate (self-test) for measuring thyroid activity. Before getting out of bed, take temperature under your arm. Should be 98.2 – 97.2 if normal. Below is sluggish (hypo) thyroid and above is overactive (hyper) thyroid.

Hyperthyroid (Graves disease)-There are two options. The first is to remove the thyroid which means you will have no way for the body to regulate calcium absorption by the bones. The second is to eliminate food additives and take kelp to encourage the thyroid to reduce its activity. Kelp has natural iodine, so the thyroid won't have to work as hard; plus eat iodine rich foods like shrimp, cabbage, broccoli and radishes. There are also herbs that can produce iodine and help keep the thyroid from over reacting: mustard powder, St. Johns wart, gentian, and bugleweed.

Hypothyroid (Low)–Symptoms include bulging eyeballs, big appetite, lots of energy and weight loss. However, this comes with side effects such as constipation, depression, diarrhea, insomnia, nervousness and palpitations of the heart. The condition may be corrected by taking high doses of the mineral Lithium, taken with two table spoons of flaxseed oil and Vitamin E. Use iodine to reduce the hypothyroid. A good source of iodine is kelp, shrimp and a thymus extract. Other important supplements include calcium, iron, selenium and zinc.

Use the iodine combo to reduce the hypothyroid condition. It should take about ten days for the thyroid to return to normal.

The answer is to detoxify the body with a multi herbal tea. Lavender should be used with the tea. However, to detox metals you should use Indian clay mixed in water as directed.

Low thyroid function known as Hypothyroidism can be traced to deficiencies in minerals, zinc, copper, selenium, amino acid tyrosine. You need pumpkin seeds, beans, almonds, soy products and fish in your diet. Drink lots of water, but not tap water, because tap water contains chlorine, which inhabits your ability to absorb iodine. Iodine is found in salts, fatty acids and sea vegetables, including Kelp, seaweed and dulse. A low thyroid condition is determined by testing body temperature. If it is consistently low, you have a thyroid problem. The temperature should be taken under the arm pit each morning for 3 consecutive days. A reading of 97.9 to 98.2 indicates a low thyroid.

Tinnitus –Take the herb oatstraw in tea. Take for 6 months before improvement. Silica can also help; purchase it under the name Avena Sativa and take as directed. Another remedy you can try is garlic oil, which should be used as if it were ear drops. Place the oil in whichever ear is infected. Also, the herbs vinpocetine, alpha lipoic acid and Beta Carnitine help to increase the circulation in the inner ears.

Toothache –Make a paste by mixing Clove oil with water and place on a cotton ball. Afterward, place the cotton ball on the infected tooth. You may substitute P73 oregano oil, which can be applied directly without making a paste.

Ulcers (On the skin) –Use a cabbage leaf as a compress.

Ulcers (stomach)–If caused by Helicobactera Pylori, the most common source of ulcers, eliminate sugar from your diet because it is a source of food for the bacteria. Also, eat yogurt, which contains lactobacillus burglarious. You should consider switching to a Mediterranean diet, which includes animal fats, apple cider vinegar, butter, cheese, fish, fruit, olive oil, red wine and vegetables.

Gut flora (bacteria) – the loss of gut flora (good bacteria) aggravates stomach ulcers. Gut flora feeds on healthy fats and cholesterol to eliminate them from the digestive tract before they enter the blood system. The loss of gut flora could lead to a gain of weight. There are a number of supplements that aid in accumulating good stomach bacteria and they include the herb licorice root.

The licorice root stimulates the mucus protective coating of the stomach and it reduces acid output. If your ulcer is the result of the bacteria, H. Pylori, licorice root can help to cure the ulcer. As a preventive measure, it is helpful to take digestive enzymes to improve digestion. The most common enzymes are contained in liquid acidophilus.

The herb curcumin (turmeric) kills the bacteria, while it also works to protect the stomach from ulcers. Another herb known for its ability to aid in the fight against ulcers is Calendula. Old time remedies, sometimes referred to as "ancient remedies" for ulcers, include: Carrots, cabbage, and celery juice. Mix in a juicer with unripened bananas and carrot juice. Drink the juice often on a daily basis for a period of two weeks.

Yet another remedy (Chinese) is a product called Wei You Pian (Fare you Gastro), which contains cabbage root and magnolia bark. Take as directed. In addition, you should take digestive enzymes, multi-vitamins and colloidal trace minerals. Other foods that are helpful in the battle against ulcers include: cabbage juice garlic, ginger, the vegetable rhubarb and the herb Plantain.

Colloidal Minerals, which are also excellent supplements; particularly because the minerals contain a key ingredient called bismuth. This helps to eliminate the H-plylori bacteria. Another helpful supplement is zinc and yet others include: Vitamin A, Vitamin C, Vitamin E and fish oil.

Urinary Tract Infections–Option 1-Drink organic cranberry juice (unsweetened) frequently for three continuous days. Drinking cranberry juice regularly prevents bacteria from attaching to the walls of the bladder. You may also use the supplement d-mannose. Other supplements to take include: a multi-vitamin, colloidal minerals and digestive enzymes.

Option 2 – 8 ounces of cranberry juice at bedtime and pipsissewa or uva ursi tincture. Drink often on a daily basis.

Option 3 – When you are affected by a urinary tract infection, make tea from dried watermelon seeds (let tea seep for 15 minutes).

Option 4 – Goldenseal tea or cornsilk tea, drink often.

Option 5 – Olive leaf capsules. Take as directed to stimulate white blood cells to destroy bacteria. Olive leaf has more antioxidants then green tea. It is an immune system activator and it is also antifungal and anti-inflammatory.

Option 6 – Make a cup or pot of tea, using the herbs juniper berry and cornsilk, which act as a disinfectant and a diuretic.

Option 7 – Take goldenrod and stinging nettles, which are both anti-bacterial herbs. These herbs may also be added to tea as a tincture.

Option 8–Take four drops of P73 oregano oil, which is anti-bacterial. Place the drops under the tongue for as long as possible, but for a minimum of five minutes before you swallow it.

Vision Problems - See Eyes.

Warts – An over the counter product, Freeze, can be effective against warts. Other remedies include covering the wart with duct tape and yet other remedies include placing a slice of potato or a piece of banana peel upon the wart. Rub a banana peel or the slice of potato on the wart a few times a day. Others include: crush aspirin and make a paste with water. Put paste on wart, not skin, and cover with a band aid after it dries, 2 times daily. Also, put a dose of apple cider vinegar on the wart each day. When the surface of the wart gets hard and scaly, it may be possible to scrape part of it away.

Another product known to be helpful against warts is Salicylic acid, which is derived from the sap from a fig tree. Silver nitrate and a caustic pencil are also helpful; both are available at a drug store.

Weight Loss –If your PH is acidic, going on a crash diet will not help you lose weight. An acidic body makes you vulnerable to gaining weight, due to an increase in the production of insulin. The increase in insulin automatically causes the body to store additional fat. It is important to remember that starvation also triggers the body to produce more insulin, however, rather than losing fat, the body will be tricked into losing muscle tissue, because the body reacts by moving into a self-preservation mode that directs it to preserve the fat as a final source of energy.

Processed food is poor in nutrition and does not satisfy hunger. Eating food that is poor in nutrition leaves a void, which causes a constant urge to eat more food, which causes a weight gain.

Supplements that may aid in losing weight:

→Hydroxyl citric acid suppresses appetite. Take as directed.

→Dark grapes (preferably with seeds) help break down fat tissue.

→For controlling weight, eat brown seaweed. It works to reduce fat tissue.

→Hot Peppers-One regimen you should try is adding hot peppers to your diet, because it increases your metabolism.

→Apple cider vinegar burns fat and helps to remove waste from cells.

→Organic coconut oil or olive oil, taken before each meal helps with the digestive tract by moving the food through the process, while either oil helps to burn fat.

→Herbal teas such as Yerbamate increase energy, while reducing the appetite.

→Coleus Forskohlii-an herb which helps the body to burn fat by working in conjunction with the thyroid.

→Hoodia (hard to find the real thing) is an appetite suppressant.

→Acai berries –The product Acai Max Cleanse is a natural cleanser derived from Acai berries. Take as directed.

→Eat eggs, which are rich in protein. They also work to keep your blood sugar low. However, diabetics should not eat the yolk of the egg.

Note: Low calcium in the blood triggers fat cells to store more fat.

Wounds-–Open wounds that linger without healing can be treated with raw refined sugar or honey, both of which provide an osmotic environment, in which no bacteria can survive. Use two tablespoons of sugar, mixed with honey. Place the mixture on the wound and surround it with Vaseline coated gauze, which essentially will create a dam. Place the sugar and honey mixture inside of the wrap. The dressing should be changed no less than every three days. It is important that you apply hydrogen peroxide on the wound between changes of the dressing.

Wounds and leg ulcers (slow healing due to poor circulation)-use calendula salve or yarrow tea. Other supplements include: Vinegar, which can be used to disinfect a wound; Chickweed, mixed with Queen Anne's laced tea and Garcinia an herb that works to burn fat.

Wrinkles – Grape seed extract and Vitamin C liquids mixed together; applied topically are good for wrinkles; they act as a skin softener. The following is helpful:

Antioxidants – Vitamin C, K and Linoleic acid (an omega 6 fatty acid), taken as supplements, makes the skin elastic and protects it against UV light damage. More importantly, the body needs alkaline blood, rather than acid blood, to prevent free radicals from depleting collagen (membrane that protects the cells). Acid blood causes the skin to appear older than the person's actual age.

Clay mask (Indian clay or bentonite clay) applied with water as a paste, may clear up various skin problems including acne, eczema and ulcers. The clay mask also helps to detoxify the liver. Many skin problems are caused by the accumulation of toxins in the body, which attempt to escape the body through the pores of the skin.

Two over the counter products that are useful in helping prevent wrinkles: Synovoderma, which should be used as directed to help in the process of replacing dead skin with fresh skin. The other product is a drink called Toki, which contains collagen, hyaluric acid, stevia and other herbs that are useful in forestalling facial aging. In conjunction, a baby's skin naturally contains an abundance of hyaluric acid; however as a person ages, hyaluric acid in the body begins to diminish. Nonetheless, hyaluric acid is necessary for the body to have excellent skin.

Yeast overgrowth–Can be controlled with Shitake mushrooms. They help the body make interferon, a natural anti-pathogen.

A product called Vitanica Yeast Arrest (suppository)–Take as directed.

Zinc fights infection and aids in DNA and RNA synthesis.

This Page Intentionally Left Blank

CHAPTER SEVEN

Tips for Women

Birth Control--Women who use birth control should eat kelp because of its iodine content.

Cyst (Ovarian)--Several possibilities exist for the creation of cysts which include the need for detoxification (see Chapter Two) to clean out the liver. An over toxified body can result in changes within the body and the skin as the body attempts to remove these toxins. Unfortunately, toxins don't make it to the skin's surface and find a home internally.

Toxins are not just in the air and water. They are also in the food we eat like pesticides, lead aluminum (pots) and mystery ingredients in processed foods.

Besides detoxifying, milk thistle can protect the liver if taken regularly. Also, the following will help: Colloidal Minerals; Oregano oil; Multi Vitamins (especially those high in Vitamins A, C and E; magnesium; black currant oil; fish oil; primrose oil and zinc.

Another factor to consider regarding ovarian cysts is consuming too much refined sugar in the diet and yet another factor is fried foods. Try to eat more organic foods like beets, carrots, and lemons, all of which help in detoxification. Eating the above mentioned as raw rather than cooked is more beneficial because when eaten raw, they provide the body with enzymes, the catalyst of our immune system.

Folic acid– reduces homocysteine levels – should be taken with B-12 and B-6. A lack of folic acid in pregnant women can lead to birth defects.

Estrogen–Estrogen is a natural hormone that is a primary fighter in the struggle to prevent bone loss, which frequently begins in women during menopause and accelerates after menopause. Use natural estrogen, natural progesterone cream and a combination of calcium and magnesium. If you don't use HRT then make sure you eat substantial amounts of fermented soy products, which contain Phytoestrogens that help to reduce hot flashes, night sweats and vaginal dryness. Soy extracts, which are available over the counter, are effective against low estrogen conditions. It is recommended that high standardized soy extract of isoflavonoids be taken. Take as directed.

Estrogen in its natural form is contained in certain foods, such as: apples, barley, brown rice, flaxseed, grapefruit, lemons, oats, oranges, whole wheat and watermelon. Estrogen is also found in some herbs, such as; carraway seed, fennel seed, oregano, parsley, rosemary, sage and tumeric.

The Chinese consume lots of foods that contain natural estrogen, which may explain why the cancer rate in Chinese women is about half of the rate of women in the United States.

It is also important to consider the possibility of too much estrogen in the body, which may be the cause of migraines, dizziness and headaches. Sleep problems can also be a factor and if you suspect this is possible, then applying progesterone cream will help keep estrogen in balance.

Reduce Estrogen related cancer–Take a self-test (NLS Female hormone saliva test). If your estrogen is high, you should eat estrogen lowering foods including: bok choy(Chinese cabbage), mustard, greens, cauliflower, cabbage, broccoli, and the mineral selenium if you are not taking recommended Colloidal Minerals (trace minerals) that contain selenium.

Hormone Imbalance--Hormone imbalance means too little of some and not enough of others. Production of hormones is the job of the endocrine system that includes the following glands: adrenal, pancreas, pituitary, testes, thymus, thyroid, and the ovaries.

A lot of hormones flow in the blood stream, including prolactin, which aids in the production of breast milk. Others include andrenocarticotrophin, a thyroid hormone that regulates fat, and sumatotrophin which is a growth hormone for the body's development. It also helps to produce estrogen, progesterone and testosterone.

Signs of hormone imbalance include moodiness, weight gain, low sex drive, poor memory, fatigue, and hot flashes. Most hormonal problems center around estrogen being too high and progesterone too low. This is a common problem for women as they grow older due to reduced production of estrogen and progesterone hormones.

If your estrogen is too high you need to supplement with bioidentical progesterone topical cream to keep progesterone in balance with the higher estrogen level.

Too much estrogen can also be the result of a high unfermented soy diet, heredity and obesity or pregnancy.

Self testing to see if an in balance exists is available. See HealthCheckUSA.com or call 1-800-929-2044.

Suggestions and supplements to take include:

→Progesterone Cream –apply at nighttime.

→Exercise – strenuous exercise activates the Human Growth Hormone.

→Amino Acids – Take Bragg's Amino Acids after dinner.

→Vitamin B-3 – helps to activate the human growth hormone (HGH).

→Herbal tea or Green tea-- anti-inflammatory herb like turmeric, garlic, onions, asparagus, curcumin. Drink often.

It is also important that you avoid sugar, carbs, processed food and high consumption of red meat.

Synthetic Hormones--Women who use synthetic hormones sometimes suffer side effects, including weight gain or bloating. There are about thirty separate side effects and they can be found in a physicians desk reference.

Pregnant women need folic acid to prevent behavior problems in newborns.

Low Libido (sex drive) **Women** –The loss of sex drive in a woman could be the result of a deficiency of the following: Coenzyme Q10, and L–Arginine (nitrate acid). The cause could also be due to a mineral or vitamin deficiency. A high potency multi-vitamin and

Colloidal Minerals can help to eliminate the deficiencies.

An herb called Maca (available in extract or capsules) used for centuries by the South Americans as a sex stimulant. Other stimulating herbs include: Yohimbe in tincture, take as directed; Kava, which relaxes blood vessels, allowing more blood flow. The herb Okakura, a seed, is a an ingredient in a lot of Aphrodisiacs. Herbs such as Triphala, Ginkgo Biloba and L-Arginine all increase circulation. Other good items are garlic, raw celery and herbal teas.

Diet is also important. Eating more good fats helps raise HDL levels and is a good source of energy. Include in your diet the following: fish oil, olive oil, canola oil, butter, fish, flaxseed oil and coconut oil. Stay away from fried foods, white flour products and sugar (white). Our current medical philosophy of a low fat and low cholesterol diet has increased in women with calcium deficiencies, low sex drives and poor vaginal lubrication.

Another good dietary consideration is raw honey, for good enzymes. It is a catalyst of the immune system and a source of energy. Eggs have Vitamin B6 and B5, which are necessary to keep hormone balanced. Nuts and celery also keep help keep the balance. Include bananas for B vitamins, potassium, enzymes and energy. Clams and oysters contain the hormone dopamine and zinc, which are necessary to initiate the sex drive.

Unfermented soy, is an "estrogen disruptor" that may inhibit cell growth and it can cause reproductive cell mutations. It contains compounds similar to estrogen that may affect the memory and judgment. Use fermented soy temp and miso because unfermented soy products contain weak estrogen hormones, which replace the body's normal and stronger hormones. Too much protein causes acid byproducts that pull calcium from the bones and afterward the byproducts enter the kidney before being excreted.

Exercise is also important because it reduces cell degeneration. Estrogen polyps, uterus fibroids, endometriosis could indicate an estrogen abundance. Take a product called Progest, which is a natural progesterone. Use as directed and combine with red clover herb as a tea.

DHEA is known as the "mother of hormones" in the fight against osteoporosis. It is important to have your blood levels checked.

After menopause, in the event that estrogen levels fall, the parathyroid gland causes a loss of calcium, while they sleep. While a person sleeps, no food is consumed, which prevents the body from receiving any calcium. During the day, the body requires substantial amounts of calcium in the blood to neutralize the loss of calcium from the bones during the hours of sleep. Consumption of dairy products that contain hormones and antibiotics, both of which are used by some farmers to increase milk production, can cause fibroids, breast cancer, ovarian cancer, acne, endometriosis and menstrual cramps (Gynecologist Christine North, MD-Women's Bodies, NY. Bantam Publishing, NY).

Women should also regularly self-massage their breasts due to the restrictions caused by wearing a bra. The massage keeps the lymph system in motion, as well as, keeping the cells (good and bad) moving. If the bad cells are either cancer cells or radical cells, keeping the lymph system moving helps starve the bad cells and helps the lymph glands aid in the destruction of the bad cells.

Morning sickness–Morning sickness can actually last all day. About thirty percent of women, who become pregnant, develop morning sickness. The cause of this phenomenon eludes explanation, but various hypothesis exist. One theory is that morning sickness coincides with increases in estrogen.

→**Vitamins B6 and B12 deficiencies**–The use of multivitamins decreases the chances of getting nausea.

→**Vitamin C (ascorbic acid)**–Excerpted from New England Journal of Medicine, October 14, 2010 page 1544 volume 363, NO. 16, By Jennifer R. Nieby MD. Vitamin C, take 400mg; Vitamin K3, take 5mg. Take both together at the same time each day for three consecutive days.

Pregnancy--Mother's breast milk is one part lactose and one part lactase. This latter enzyme is important in the development of an infant's nervous system since the nerves are wrapped in a myelin sheath. This enzyme is only available in breast milk since infant's livers are not developed enough to convert lactose to lactase.

High sugar intake and refined carbs and lack of exercise can elevate blood sugars.

Vegetarians have trouble making good iron levels and breast feeding depletes iron supplies. Nursing mothers need a good dietary supply of iron. Iron in meat is the best absorbed. Pregnant women need the following: Calorie, protein, calcium, iron, zinc, B vitamin, multi vitamin, 74 trace mineral supplement, and folic acid for red blood cell production. See full list of vitamins to follow.

Low salt diet (to reduce water retention)-- no junk food no fried foods, no white sugar or white flour products; they are dead foods (no nutrition). You also need high fiber for good bowel movements combined with digestive enzymes like yogurt or sauerkraut. A good herbal tea for nutrients and black raspberry tea is an old folk remedy for strong uterus and easy labor. Also, no pharmaceutical drugs.

Necessary vitamins and minerals are as follows: keep in mind that if you are breast feeding, it puts an even greater demand on nutrition by 25%.

Vitamin A--usually obtained by diet; Vitamin D; chromium; Vitamin E, copper; Vitamin K, usually obtained from diet; Vitamin B1; iodine; Vitamin B2; iron; Vitamin B3; magnesium; Vitamin B5; Manganese; Vitamin B6; Molybdenum; Vitamin B12; Phosphorus; Vitamin C; selenium; Folic acid; sodium, usually obtained from diet; Boitin; Potassium, usually obtained from diet; Choline; zinc; Inositol, essential fatty acids; PABA (Para-aminobenzoic acid); bioflavonoids and Calcium.

Vaginal dryness–Two over the counter products that are helpful for this condition are: Vaginal Estriol and KY jelly.

Personal Notes: